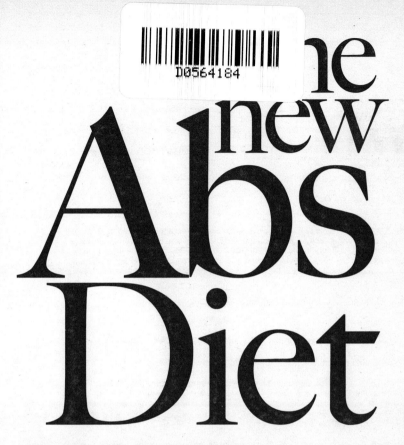

The new Abs Diet

The Six-Week Plan to
Flatten Your Stomach
and Keep You Lean for Life

DAVID ZINCZENKO

Editorial Director of **Men'sHealth**

WITH TED SPIKER

RODALE

This edition first published 2010 by Rodale
an imprint of Pan Macmillan, a division of Macmillan Publishers Limited
First published in paperback 2006 © Rodale Inc
Pan Macmillan, 20 New Wharf Road, London N1 9RR
Basingstoke and Oxford
Associated companies throughout the world
www.panmacmillan.com

ISBN 978-1-9057-44-59-6

1 3 5 7 9 8 6 4 2

A CIP catalogue record for this book is available from the British Library.

Printed and bound in Great Britain by CPI Mackays, Chatham ME5 8TD

This book is intended as a reference volume only, not as a medical manual. The information given here is designed to help you make informed decisions about your health. It is not intended as a substitute for any treatment that you may have been prescribed by your doctor. If you suspect you have a medical problem, we urge you to seek competent medical help.

Mention of specific companies, organizations or authorities in this book does not imply endorsement of the publisher, nor does mention of specific companies, organizations or authorities in the book imply that they endorse the book.
Addresses, websites and telephone numbers given in this book were correct at the time of going to press.

Some portions of this book have appeared previously in *Men's Health* magazine.

Visit **www.panmacmillan.com** to read more about all our books and to buy them. You will also find features, author interviews and news of any author events, and you can sign up for e-newsletters so that you're always first to hear about our new releases.

RODALE
LIVE YOUR WHOLE LIFE

Contents

Acknowledgments

MY DEEPEST THANKS TO the extraordinarily talented, hardworking and dedicated people who have supported me, encouraged me and inspired me. In particular:

Steve Murphy, who over the past 10 years turned Rodale Inc. into an international publishing powerhouse by having the insight and courage to put editorial quality first.

The Rodale family, especially our new CEO Maria Rodale, without whom none of this would be possible.

Jeremy Katz, my editor, who saw my vision for *The Abs Diet*, pushed me to make it the best I could, and talked me down off more than one ledge during its creation.

Steve Perrine, the wisest consigliere any boss could ever have.

The entire *Men's Health* editorial staff, the smartest and hardest-working group of writers, editors, researchers, designers and photo directors in the industry. In the future, when people talk about the glory days of men's magazine publishing, they will be talking about you.

My brother, Eric, whose relentless teasing shamed me into taking better care of myself.

My mother, Janice, who raised the two of us nearly single-handedly. Your strength and kindness guide my every action.

To my dad, Bohdan, who left this world way too early. I wish you were still here.

And to my stepmother, Mickey. Thanks for your guidance and support.

For everyone who has taken up arms in the
battle against obesity. Today we begin
winning the fight...

WELCOME TO THE NEW ABS DIET!

There's no better time to make over your body than right now.

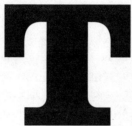

HE ABS DIET LAUNCHED IN THE United Kingdom five years ago. Since then, tens of thousands of people here have used the programme to lose weight, shape up, dramatically improve their health and, yes, turn their bellies as flat and hard as the business end of a cricket bat.

But there's more work to do. While much has changed in our world in five years' time, much remains the same – or has got worse. Obesity continues to spread like a pandemic. It has reached crisis proportions in the US, where it has overtaken smoking as the leading cause of premature heart attacks. And things are getting nearly as bad in England, where almost 1 in 4 adults is currently obese. Unless more Britons adopt healthier eating and exercise habits, the number of overweight or obese adults will rise to 9 in 10 by 2050, according to National Health Service estimates.

We must halt those expanding waistlines. Fortunately, we know even more about exercise and nutritional science than we did five years ago and as a result the Abs Diet is more relevant than ever before. While so many diets have fallen off the radar screen, the Abs Diet has stood the test of time because it's not based on fads or gimmicks or fleeting promises. It's grounded in sound principles of nutrition and the latest clinical science.

And it's easy to follow.

Look, recent studies on human nutrition in both the US and UK point to one of the simplest ways to clean up your diet and shed significant pounds: Eliminate added sugars. The average American consumes 80 grams of added sugar every day; in the UK, young men average 96 grams daily, mostly from drinks, sugar added to foods, and sweets. (That's eating 77 pounds of sugar in a year!) By simply avoiding foods that contain added sugar, you're diet will instantly become healthier and you'll lose weight. What's more, 2009 research from the University of Nottingham found that you can burn 50 per cent more fat during a workout simply by eating healthier foods. Imagine that, you can double the effectiveness of exercise by fueling your body right! And even more recent research supports the power of regular exercise to reverse bad habits and the health problems they trigger. A study reported in the *British Medical Journal* in 2009 suggests that starting an exercise programme from scratch in middle age can make you as healthy as someone who's been exercising regularly for years. In fact, your reduction in mortality risk will be comparable to quitting smoking!

The new Abs Diet is loaded with tools to help you reach your weight-loss, fitness and health goals. We've packed this new edition with more useful tips and advice as well as bonus chapters on motivation offering 10 ways to stick to your diet and fitness plan, strategies to get the most out of cardio machine workouts and burn fat faster, and an all-new abs-specific workout that'll turn your six pack into an eight pack! Try this amazingly effective programme for eight weeks, and see fantastic results.

Seeing the Abs Diet do so well in the United Kingdom has been one of the great pleasures of my life. Thank you for purchasing a copy and embarking on this journey. I'm confident that this programme will help you to reach your weight-loss and fitness goals – and finally reveal those abs!

David Zinczenko
December, 2009

Introduction

YOU HAVE ABS.
YES, YOU.
The Plan That Will Turn Your Fat into Muscle

WHEN YOU THINK OF ABS, you may think of Brad Pitt or Janet Jackson. You may think of magazine covers and underwear commercials. You may think of six-packs, washboards and a stomach so tight that you could bounce a marble off it. Your cynical side may also think of airbrushing, starvation diets and an exercise regime so time-consuming it would violate health and safety laws. Abs, you assume, are reserved for athletes, for models, for bodybuilders, for trainers, for rappers, for genetic freaks, for the liposuctioned, and for people who would classify celery as a dessert.

Your conclusion: you have a better chance of scaling Mount Everest in a swimsuit than you do of getting great abs.

As the editor-in-chief of *Men's Health* magazine, I know that you – no matter how big your belly, how many diets you've tried or how tempting the Everest swimsuit challenge sounds – can develop great abs. See, I analyse health and fitness information the way brokers analyse the market. It's my job to find the fastest, best and smartest ways for you to make tremendous gains in your most important investment: your body. So when I think about abs, the only thing I think about is this: how you can get them.

I understand the struggle. You look down, see a jelly mould implanted in your gut, and figure that your days of having a flat stomach vanished the day you left school. But in a way, you really shouldn't think of your abs as being extinct. Think of your abs as the third cousins you met at a past family reunion. You remember seeing them, so you have a vague memory of what they look like, but it's been so long that you really don't have a clue where they are now. Well, even if it's been decades since you've made any kind of contact with them, the physiological fact remains: you have abs.

The Abs Diet is going to help you find them.

At a time when more than two in five adults in the UK are overweight, and a further one in five is obese, and when weight-loss news garners as much front-page attention as celebrity scandals (well, almost as much), there's never been a more critical time to focus on your weight, your shape and your health. I know that some critics will see a chiselled midsection as the modern symbol of vanity, but developing a six-pack is more than just a way to support the mirror industry.

Abs are the contemporary badge of fitness.

They're the ultimate predictor of your health.

And since flat stomachs boost sex appeal, they represent the one part of your body that has the same power of seduction over both men and women.

Depending on where you fall on the body-shape scale, there's a good chance you've searched for your abs before. Maybe you've failed on previous weight-loss attempts, and maybe you've yo-yoed more than a toy shop. I know what you've gone through – I've talked to and heard from thousands of people who have shared their weight-loss success stories with *Men's Health*. But I also know what you've gone through because I, too, know what it's like to feel fat.

As a latchkey kid growing up in the early '80s, I made every mistake in the book. I ate fast food instead of smart food. I played video games when I should've been playing outside. By the time I reached 14, I was carrying 95 kg/15 st of torpid teenage tallow on my 1.77 m/5 ft 10 in frame. I wanted to be built like a basketball player, but instead I was built like the basketball. And I paid for it with a steady bombardment of humiliation. My older brother, Eric, would invite friends to our house just to watch me eat lunch. 'Don't disturb the big animal,' he'd tell his friends. 'It's feeding.'

Like most kids, I learned my health habits from my parents, particularly my father. He was more than 45 kg/7 st overweight for most of his adult life. Over time, he developed hypertension and diabetes, had a minor heart attack, and would have to stop at the top of a short flight of stairs just to catch his breath. A massive stroke ended his life at the age of 52. My father died because he ignored many signals of failing health – especially the fat that padded his gut.

But I got lucky. When I left school, I joined the Naval Reserve, where the tenets of fitness were pounded into me, day after day after day. Soon after I graduated from college, I joined *Men's Health* and learned the importance of proper nutrition and – just as important – the danger of carrying around too much fat in your gut.

Belly fat – the fat that pushes your waist out – is the most dangerous fat on your body. And it's one of the reasons why the Abs Diet emphasizes losing belly fat – because doing so means you'll live longer. Belly fat is classified as visceral fat; that means it is located behind your abdominal wall and surrounds your internal organs. Because it's on a fast track to your heart and other important organs, visceral fat is the fat that can kill you. Just consider one University of Alabama–Birmingham study in which researchers used seven different measurements to determine a person's risks of cardiovascular disease. They concluded that the amount of visceral fat the subjects carried was the single best predictor of heart disease risk.

Whether you want to change your body to improve your health, your looks, your athletic performance or your sex appeal, the Abs Diet offers you a simple promise: if you follow this plan, you will transform your body so that you can accomplish each and every one of those goals. As a bonus, the Abs Diet will do something more than just enhance your life; the Abs Diet is going to save it.

When you think of all you have to gain with the Abs Diet, it becomes apparent what's wrong with most diet plans out there: they're all about losing. When you consider the West's obesity epidemic, losing weight is an admirable goal. But I think there's a fundamental psychological reason why many of these diets fail: there's no motivation in losing. Most of us don't like to lose. We don't like to lose a round of golf. We don't like to lose on the stock market. We don't like to lose our looks. We don't like to lose anything. In a way, we don't even like losing weight, because we've all been force-fed the notion that bigger is better. Instead, we're programmed to gain. We want to gain fitness. We want to gain strength. We want to add to our life, not subtract from it. We're empire builders. We want to win – and see our results. So consider the Abs Diet a shift in the way you think about your body and about weight loss. This programme concentrates on what you can gain and how you can gain it. As a result of what you'll gain from this programme – abs, muscle tone, better health, a great sex life (more on that later) – you'll effortlessly strip away fat from your body and change your body shape for ever.

No diet plan would work without good nutrition, so that, of course, is the major focus of the Abs Diet. You'll not only learn what to eat; you'll learn how to eat to make your body burn fat furiously, as well as how to make sure that you can control the cravings that threaten to add girth to your gut. The focus of the plan revolves around – but does not restrict you to – 12 'Powerfoods' that are among the best sources for protein, fibre and all the other ingredients and nutrients that help fight fat. When you build your diet around these foods, you will build a new body in the process. But we've taken this weight-loss plan to a whole other level. While nutrition remains a principal component of most diets, too many programmes out there focus solely on how to change your eating habits – cut carbs, add cabbage soup, eat at Subway twice a day. Those programmes fail to recognize a crucial component of weight control: the fact that our bodies have their own natural fat-burning mechanism...

Muscle.

Building just a few kilograms of muscle in your body is the physiological equivalent of kicking fat out of the door and telling it to never come back again. Muscle exponentially speeds up the fat-busting process: half a kilo/1 lb of muscle requires your body to burn up to 50 extra calories a day just to maintain that muscle. Now think about what happens if you add a mere 2.75 kg/6 lb of muscle over the course of a diet programme. It'll take your body up to 300 extra calories a day just to feed that muscle; essentially, you'll burn off an extra ½ kg/1 lb of fat every 10 days without doing a thing (and that's not even including the gains you can make by changing your diet). When you combine exercise with the foods that most promote muscle growth, the ones that keep you full, and the ones that give your body a well-balanced supply of nutrients, you'll be in the sweet spot, doing what this plan is all about.

You'll turn your fat into muscle.

Does that mean the Abs Diet is going to make you burly, bulky, muscle-bound, or governor of California? Not at all. The Abs Diet and the accompanying Abs Diet Workout emphasize leanness and muscle tone – not big, bulky muscles.

Going back to that important investment, you can think about muscle as your compound interest. If you've ever taken a basic economics course, then you understand how compound interest works: if you invest £100 in a high-yield fund and add a little more every month, over time that investment will grow and grow to half a million pounds or more. But you'll have

FOREWORD: DIET IS A FOUR-LETTER WORD

In all honesty, I hated to even call this book a 'diet' book. That's because the word *diet* has been twisted around to mean something you follow temporarily – you 'go on a diet'. But if you 'go on' a diet, you eventually have to 'go off' it. And that's why most diets are really, really bad for you.

Most diets are about eating less food or about restricting you to certain kinds of food. Most of them work in the short term, because if you reduce your calorie intake, your body starts to burn itself off in order to keep itself alive. Hey presto, you lose weight. But here's the problem: the first thing your body does when it's short of calories is to dump the body tissue that takes the most calories to maintain. That's muscle. So on a low-calorie diet, your body burns away muscle and tries to store fat. Sure, you'll lose weight, and you'll eventually start losing fat as well. But when you 'go off' your diet, you'll start to put weight back on. And guess what kind of weight you'll gain? Pure fat. Because you've taught your body a harsh lesson: it has to be on the lookout for potential low-calorie periods in the future, so it had better store fat just in case. You've also used up valuable calorie-burning muscle, so you're likely to end up fatter than you were before your diet. That's why people who try diet after diet not only don't lose weight, they gain it.

The Abs Diet isn't a wham-bam-thank-you-ma'am approach to weight management. Oh, you'll lose weight, and you'll lose it fast. But you'll lose fat, not muscle. And you'll keep that weight off for life. You'll follow the tenets of the Abs Diet for life, too, because it's about eating lots and lots of great food in smart ways. So enjoy the Abs Diet. But let's keep that little four-letter word between us, OK?

invested only a fraction of the money yourself. Compound interest is what allows you to make the most dramatic financial gains. It's the same concept with your body. Invest in a little additional muscle in the next 6 weeks – through eating the right foods and following a muscle-building, fat-burning exercise plan – and you'll have invested in a lean and strong body that can last a lifetime, because your new muscle will continually break down fat to stay alive.

I'm passionate about this plan because I know it works. I've seen it work, and so will you. During the course of this 6-week plan, you can lose up to 9 kg/20 lb of fat (much of it in the first couple of weeks, and from your belly first) and gain 1.8 to 2.75 kg/ 4 to 6 lb of lean muscle. But the biggest thing you'll notice is that you'll have significantly changed the shape of your body. Some of you will have even more dramatic results (see page 48 for the story of Bill Stanton, who lost 13.6 kg/2 st 2 lb on the diet and cut his body fat percentage in half). The Abs Diet includes all three components to a successful body-transforming programme: nutrition, exercise and the motivational principles to follow through. I've designed this programme to make it easy to stick to, even if you've tried and failed with diets in the past. It's easy to follow because:

▶ Every component of the diet and exercise plan is quick, simple and flexible enough so that you can easily work it into your life.

▶ Every goal is attainable.

▶ Every principle is supported by well-respected scientific research.

The Abs Diet will change the way you think about your body. It's the first plan to count not just the calories your body takes in but the calories your body burns off as well. Using the most cutting-edge nutrition and exercise research, the Abs Diet will show you how to retrain your body to burn fat faster and more efficiently – even while you sleep – and to focus your meals around the foods that inspire your body to keep those calorie-burning fires stoked. The Abs Diet isn't about counting calories; it's about making your calories count.

Throughout the book, I'll take you through the principles of the Abs Diet and show you how to follow the 6-week plan. I'll also explain the exercise programme (which doesn't have to start until the third week) and give you instructions on how to perform the exercises and how to make the meals. (Don't worry – if you can operate a blender, you can cook up our Powerfood feasts.)

To keep you motivated, I've included the stories of real-life men and women who credit the Abs Diet with changing their bodies and their lives – not to mention the size of their trousers.

THE ABS DIET CHEAT SHEET

 **HIS AT-A-GLANCE GUIDE** summarizes the principles of the Abs Diet: the 6-week plan to flatten your stomach and keep you lean for life.

SUBJECT	GUIDELINE
Number of meals	Six a day, spaced relatively evenly throughout the day. Eat snacks 2 hours before larger meals.
The **ABS DIET POWER 12**	Base most of your meals on these 12 groups of foods. Every meal should have at least two foods from the list.

Almonds and other nuts
Beans and pulses
Spinach and other green vegetables

Dairy (skimmed milk, fat-free or low-fat yogurt and cheese)
Instant hot oat cereal (unsweetened, unflavoured)
Eggs
Turkey and other lean meats

Peanut butter
Olive oil
Wholegrain breads and cereals
Extra-protein (whey) powder
Raspberries and other berries

SUBJECT	GUIDELINE
Secret weapons	Each of the ABS DIET POWER 12 has been chosen in part for its stealthy, healthy secret weapons – the nutrients that will help power up your natural fat burners, protect you from illness and injury, and keep you lean and fit for life!
Nutritional ingredients to emphasize	Protein, monounsaturated and polyunsaturated fats, fibre, calcium.
Nutritional ingredients to limit	Refined carbohydrates (or carbs with high glycaemic index), saturated fats, trans fats, high-fructose corn syrup, glucose syrup, modified starch.
Alcohol	Limit yourself to two or three drinks per week, to maximize the benefits of the Abs Diet plan.
Ultimate power food	Smoothies. The combination of the calcium and protein in milk, yogurt and whey powder, combined with the fibre in oats and fruit, makes them one of the more filling and easy options in the diet. Drink them regularly.
Cheating	One meal a week, eat anything you want.
Exercise programme	Optional for the first 2 weeks. Weeks 3 to 6 incorporate a 20-minute, full-body workout 3 days a week. Emphasis is on strength training, brisk walking and some abdominal work.
At-home workout	Gym workouts and at-home workouts are both detailed to excuse-proof your fitness plan.
Abdominal workout	At the beginning of two of your strength-training workouts. One exercise for each of the five different parts of your abs.

Chapter I

STRIP AWAY FAT, STRIP AWAY TROUBLE

Six Ways a Flat Stomach Will Dramatically Improve
How You Look, Feel and Live

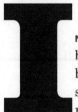N GYMS, PLAYING FIELDS, BEACHES AND bedrooms across the country, our bodies are constantly being measured. And in dressing room mirrors and on bathroom scales, we're constantly measuring ourselves. But let's set aside those vanity measurements and concentrate on measuring ourselves by a different set of criteria – the number of fat cells we're carrying.

The average person has about 30 billion fat cells; each of them is filled with greasy substances called lipids. When you pump doughnuts, chips and Mars bars into your system, those fat cells can expand – up to 1,000 times their original size. But a fat cell can get only so big; once it reaches its physical limit, it starts to behave like a long-running sitcom. It creates spin-offs, leaving you with two or more fat cells for the price of one. Only problem: fat cells have a no-return policy. Once you have a fat cell, you're stuck with it. So as you grow fatter and double the number of fat cells in your body, you also double the difficulty you'll have losing the lipids inside them.

Many of us tend to store fat around our waists, and that's where the health dangers of excess weight begin. Abdominal fat doesn't just sit there and do nothing; it's active. It functions like a separate organ, releasing substances that can be harmful to your body. For instance, it releases free fatty acids that impair your ability to break down the hormone insulin (too much insulin in your system can lead to diabetes). Fat also secretes substances that increase your risk of heart attacks and strokes, as well as the stress hormone cortisol (high levels of cortisol are also associated with diabetes and obesity as well as with high blood pressure). Abdominal fat bears the blame for many health problems because it resides within striking distance of your heart, liver and other organs – pressing on them, feeding them poisons and messing with their daily function.

Now take the person with a six-pack. He's the icon of strength and good health. He's lean; he's strong; he looks good in clothes; he looks good without clothes. Defined abs, in many ways, have defined fitness. But they define something else: they're the hallmark of a person who's in control of his body and, as such, in control of his health.

While some people may think that working towards abs of armour is shallower than a paddling pool, there's nothing wrong with striving for a six-pack. Of course, defined abs make you look good – and make others feel good about the way you look, too.

(Take heed, men: in one survey, 32 per cent of women said that abs are the muscles most likely to make them melt; the next closest was biceps at 17 per cent.) And for good reason: when you have abs, you're telling the world that you're a disciplined, motivated, confident and healthy person – and hence a desirable partner. And sometimes a little vanity can be good for your health: in a recent Canadian study of more than 8,000 people, researchers found that over 13 years, those with the weakest abdominal muscles had a death rate more than twice as high of those with the strongest midsections. Such research upholds the notion that strong abs do more than turn heads at the beach. In fact, your abdominal muscles control more of your body than you may realize – and have just as much substance as show. In short, here are my top six reasons why striving for a six-pack is going to make your life better.

Abs Will Help You Live Longer

STUDY AFTER STUDY shows that the people with the largest waist sizes have the most risk of life-threatening disease. The evidence couldn't be more convincing. According to the American National Institutes of Health, a waistline larger than 102 cm/40 in for men signals significant risk of heart disease and diabetes. The Canadian Heart Health Surveys, published in 2001, looked at 9,913 people aged 18 to 74 and concluded that, for maximum health, a man needs to keep his waist size at no more than 87 cm/35 in (a little less for younger men, a little more for older ones). When your waist grows larger than 89 cm/35 in, you're at higher risk of developing two or more risk factors for heart disease. And when researchers examined data from the American Physicians' Health Study that has tracked 22,701 male doctors since 1982, they found that men whose waists measured more than 94 cm/36.8 in had a significantly elevated risk of myocardial infarction, or heart attack, in which an area of the heart muscle dies or is permanently damaged by a lack of bloodflow. Men with the biggest bellies were at 60 per cent higher risk. Now the really scary part: the average British man's waist size is now 102.5 cm/37 in. The recent National UK Sizing Survey revealed that average measurements around women's midriffs have increased by 17 cm/6½ in in a little over 50 years. Men's bodies are thought to have inflated by a similar proportion over the same period.

Of course, abs don't guarantee you a get-out-of-hospital-free card, but studies show that by developing a strong abdominal section, you'll reduce body fat and significantly cut the risk factors associated with many diseases, not just heart disease. For example, the incidence of cancer among obese patients is 33 per

---

ABS DIET SUCCESS STORY

'I LOST 12 KG/26 LB IN 6 WEEKS!'

Name: Paul McComb

Age: 28

Height: 1.75 m/5'9"

Starting weight: 82 kg/12 st 12 lb

Six weeks later: 70 kg/11 st

Once Paul McComb left college and gained some weight, he figured that extra heft was his to keep for life. But when he walked into a fitness centre and stepped on some scales that told him how much he weighed (82 kg/ 12 st 12 lb) and how much he should weigh (70 kg/11 st), something changed: his attitude.

So McComb went on the Abs Diet – and lost 12 kg/26 lb.

He made significant changes by doing such things as eliminating the four or five daily Cokes and skipping the midnight crisps. He says the transition was easy because the Abs Diet allowed him to eat plenty – six times a day, in fact.

cent higher than among lean ones, according to a Swedish study. The World Health Organization estimates that up to one-third of cancers of the colon, kidney and digestive tract are caused by being overweight and inactive. And having an excess of fat around your middle is especially dangerous. See, cancer is caused by mutations that occur in cells as they divide. Fat tissue in your abdomen spurs your body to produce hormones that prompt your cells to divide. More cell division means more opportunities for cell mutations, which means more cancer risk.

A lean waistline also heads off another of our most pressing health problems – diabetes. Currently, 1.3 million Britons have been diagnosed with adult-onset diabetes, and many more go undiagnosed. Fat, especially tummy fat, bears the blame. There's a misconception that diabetes comes only from eating too much

'With the eating six times a day, I didn't feel like snacking on crisps,' he reports. 'I used to not eat at all during the day; then I'd come home, eat dinner, and have crisps in the evening. When I started eating all day, it was like, holy cow, I just wasn't as hungry.'

McComb says the key to his success was planning meals around the Abs Diet Powerfoods, so he wasn't tempted by vending machines and snack bars. He'd eat turkey on multigrain bread for lunch, have wholewheat pasta or chicken for dinner, and snack on peanut butter and chocolate milk. He was happy that he didn't have to count calories, watch carbs or give up the foods he loves. 'Understanding the Powerfoods concept and how these foods work together helped me eat – a lot – and still watch the weight come off.'

McComb, who did the Abs Diet Workout at home with 9-kg/20-lb dumbbells, says he'll always incorporate the principles of the Abs Diet into his lifestyle. 'I feel a lot better now. I feel more confident because I set a goal for myself and I actually achieved it. Even my skin is a bit clearer. I find I'm getting better sleep, I'm waking up more rested, and the bags under my eyes are going away. Everything seems to be that much better in my life. I'm sure some of my friends are sick of hearing how much weight I lost.'

refined sugar, like the kind in chocolate and ice cream. But people contract diabetes after years of eating high-carbohydrate foods that are easily converted into sugar – foods like white bread, pasta and mashed potatoes. Scoffing down a basket of bread and a bowl of pasta can do the same thing to your body that a carton of ice cream does: flood it with sugar calories. The calories you can't burn are what converts into fat cells that pad your gut and leaves you with a disease that, if untreated, can lead to impotence, blindness, heart attacks, strokes, amputation and death. And that, my friend, can really ruin your day.

Upper-body obesity is also the most significant risk factor for obstructive sleep apnoea, a condition in which the soft tissue in the back of your throat collapses during sleep, blocking your airway. When that happens, your brain signals you to wake up and to start breathing again. As you nod off once more, the same thing happens, and it can continue hundreds of times during the night – making you chronically groggy and unable to get the rest your body needs. (You won't remember waking up over and over again; you'll just wonder why 8 hours of sleep left you dragging.) Fat's role is that it can impede muscles that inflate and ventilate the lungs, forcing you to work harder to get enough air. When Australian researchers studied 313 patients with severe obesity, they found that 62 per cent of them with a waist circumference of 124.5 cm/49 in or more had a serious sleep disturbance and that 28 per cent of obese patients with smaller waists (89 to 124.5 cm/35 to 49 in) had sleep problems. Being overweight also puts you at risk of a lot of other conditions that rob you of a good night's rest, including asthma and gastro-esophageal reflux. When Dutch researchers studied nearly 6,000 men, they found that even those whose waistlines measured a relatively modest 94 to 102 cm/37 to 40 in had a significantly increased risk of respiratory problems, such as wheezing, chronic coughing and shortness of breath. All of this can create an ugly cycle: abdominal fat leads to poor sleep. Poor sleep means you drag through your day. Sluggish and tired, your body craves some quick energy, so you snack on some high-calorie junk food. That extra junk food leads to more abdominal fat, which leads to . . . well, you get the picture.

I could fill this whole book with evidence, but I'm going to boil it down to one sentence: a smaller waist equals fewer health risks.

Abs Will Improve Your Sex Life

WOMEN CLAIM THE GREATEST sex organ is the brain; men say it's approximately 1 m/3 ft due south. So let's say we split the geographic difference and focus on what's really central to a good sex life.

You know the old phrase 'It's not the size of the ship; it's the motion of the ocean'? Well, take that to heart. We can't improve upon what God gave you (though the Abs Diet may actually somewhat increase the size of a guy's manhood – more on that in a bit), but we can rebuild your body to maximize the rocking and rolling that goes on below deck. Consider how the following side benefits can help you pull that ship into harbour.

Increased stamina. The thrusting power you generate during sex doesn't come from your legs; it comes from your core. Strong abdominal and lower-back muscles give you the stamina and strength to try new positions, stay steady in old ones and maintain the motion control that's important for your staying power – and your partner's pleasure.

Better erections. It's no secret that upwards of 2 million men in Britain have some kind of erectile dysfunction (roughly 10 per cent of the male population). Though many things can cause it, one of the major causes is purely a matter of traffic control. Artery-clogging cheeseburgers don't discriminate, so when you're overweight, the gunk that gums up the blood vessels leading to your heart and brain also gums up the vessels that lead to your genitals. Plaque forms on the inside of your arteries, narrowing the passageways that blood must follow. Think of 12 lanes of traffic bottlenecking into one. Your blood vessels can become so clogged in your pelvic area that a sufficient supply of blood can't get through to form an erection. You don't need to have studied calculus to understand this equation: increased fat equals decreased bloodflow. Decreased bloodflow equals softer (or no) erections. Softer (or no) erections equals 'This stinks' squared. (By the way, clogged blood vessels have the same effect on women, leading to decreased lubrication, sensitivity and sexual pleasure.)

Increased length. When it comes to a man and his privates, fat is his body's side-view mirror: objects appear smaller than actual size. The length of the average man's penis is about 8 cm/3 in flaccid, but the fatter he is, the smaller he'll look. That's because the fat at the base of a man's abdomen covers up the base of his penis. Losing just 6.8 kg/15 lb of fat will add up to 1 cm/½ inch to the length of a man's member. No, Little Elvis is not technically growing, but decreasing the fat that surrounds it will allow all a guy's got to actually show.

Abs Will Keep You Safe from Harm

IN SCHOOL, YOU were taught the story of the Great Fire of London, and how a small spark in a baker's shop resulted in some 13,000 houses being destroyed. That tragedy happened at a time when most urban housing was built with wood. Today, such a disaster is unthinkable. It's unthinkable because the infrastructure of today's cities is built with steel – steel that stands up to fire, to earthquakes, to hurricanes.

Think of your midsection as your body's infrastructure. You

don't want a core made of dry, brittle wood or straw. You want one made of solid steel, one that will give you a layer of protection that tummy fat never could.

Consider a US Army study that linked powerful abdominal muscles to injury prevention. After giving 120 artillery soldiers the standard army fitness test of sit-ups, press-ups and a 3.2 km/2-mile run, researchers tracked their lower-body injuries (such as lower-back pain and Achilles tendonitis) during a year

BABY, BABY, WHERE DID OUR LUNCH GO?

Your last meal didn't end up just in your gut. After a meal, your body begins to apportion the calories to nutrient-hungry organs, growing muscles and, yes, your tummy. Dr Michael Jenson, a professor of medicine in the division of endocrinology, diabetes and metabolism at the Mayo Clinic, calculated this breakdown of how your body processes food.

10 per cent to the kidneys. Kidneys work to make sure the blood is balanced with the right amounts of water and nutrients.

5–10 per cent to the heart. The heart gets most of its energy from fat, which provides more long-term energy for the hardworking heart than glucose can.

23 per cent to the liver, pancreas, spleen and adrenal glands. After the liver pulls out nutrients, it stores excess calories as glycogen.

25 per cent to muscles. Muscles require a constant source of energy just to maintain their mass, so the more muscle you have, the more calories you burn.

10 per cent to the brain. Glucose is brain fuel. It can't be stored long term, which is why people often feel faint if they skip a meal.

10 per cent to thermogenesis. The simple act of breaking down the food you just ate takes up one-tenth of your calories.

2–3 per cent to fat cells. Your fat cells grow and eventually divide as more and more calories are deposited.

10 per cent to no one knows where. Your body's a big place, and some calories go unaccounted for.

of field training. The 29 men who cranked out the most sit-ups (73 in 2 minutes) were five times less likely to suffer lower-body injuries than the 31 who barely notched 50. But that's not the most striking element. The men who performed well in the

FAT'S DOMINOES

Overweight people are:

▶ 50 per cent more likely to develop heart disease (obese: up to 100 per cent)

▶ Up to 360 per cent more likely to develop diabetes (obese: up to 1,020 per cent)

▶ 16 per cent more likely to die of a first heart attack (obese: 49 per cent)

▶ Roughly 50 per cent more likely to have total cholesterol above 6 mmol/L (obese: up to 122 per cent)

▶ 50 per cent more likely to have erectile dysfunction (obese: 200 per cent)

▶ 14 per cent less attractive to the opposite sex (obese: 43 per cent)

▶ Likely to spend 37 per cent more a year at the pharmacy (obese: 105 per cent)

▶ Likely to stay 19 per cent longer in hospital (obese: 49 per cent)

▶ 20 per cent more likely to have asthma (obese: 50 per cent)

▶ Up to 31 per cent more likely to die of any cause (obese: 62 per cent)

▶ 19 per cent more likely to die in a car crash (obese: 37 per cent)

▶ 120 per cent more likely to develop stomach cancer (obese: 330 per cent)

▶ Up to 90 per cent more likely to develop gallstones (obese: up to 150 per cent)

▶ 590 per cent more likely to develop oesophageal cancer (obese: 1,520 per cent)

▶ 35 per cent more likely to develop kidney cancer (obese: 70 per cent)

▶ 14 per cent more likely to have osteoarthritis (obese: 34 per cent)

▶ 70 per cent more likely to develop high blood pressure (obese: up to 170 per cent)

press-ups and 3.2 km/2-mile run enjoyed no such protection – suggesting that upper-body strength and cardiovascular endurance had little effect on keeping bodies sound. It was abdominal strength that offered the protection. Unlike any other muscles in your body, a strong core affects the functioning of the entire body. Whether you ski, sail, wrestle with the kids or fool around with a partner, your abs are the most essential muscles for keeping you from injury. The stronger they are, the stronger – and safer – you are.

Abs Will Strengthen Your Back

I HAD A FRIEND who put his back out maybe two or three times a year. He always did it in the simplest way – sleeping a little awkwardly or getting out of a chair too quickly. One time, he put it out reaching into the back seat of his car to get something his young daughter had dropped. The pain once stabbed him so badly that he collapsed to the ground while he was standing at a urinal. (Go ahead. Imagine that.) His problem wasn't that he had a bad back; it was that he had weak abs. If he had trained them regularly, he could've kept himself from being one of the millions of men who suffer from back pain every year. (And yes, he started the Abs Diet Workout a year ago, and within weeks his back pain virtually disappeared.)

Since most back pain is related to weak muscles in your trunk, maintaining a strong midsection can help resolve many back issues. The muscles that crisscross your midsection don't function in isolation; they weave through your torso like a spider's web, even attaching to your spine. When your abdominal muscles are weak, the muscles in your buttocks (your glutes) and along the backs of your legs (your hamstrings) have to compensate for the work your abs should be doing. The effect, besides promoting bad company morale for the muscles picking up the slack, is that it destabilizes the spine and eventually leads to back pain and strain – or even more serious back problems.

Abs Will Limit Your Aches and Pains

AS YOU AGE, it's common to experience some joint pain – most likely in your knees, but maybe around your feet and ankles, too. But the source of that pain might not be weak joints; it might be weak abs – especially if you're any kind of athlete, from the serious golfer to the I-pull-my-groin-every-time park football player. When you're playing sports, your abdominal muscles help stabilize your body during start-and-stop movements, like changing direction on the football pitch or tennis court. If you have weak abdominal muscles, your joints absorb all the force from those movements. It's kind of like trampoline physics. Jump in the centre, and the mat will absorb your weight and bounce you back in the air. Jump towards the side of the trampoline, where the mat meets the frame, and you'll bust the springs. Your body is sort of like a trampoline, with your abs as the centre of the mat and your joints as the supports that hold the mat to the frame. If your abs are strong enough to absorb some shock, you'll function well. If they're not, the force puts far more pressure on your joints than they were built to withstand.

Similar protection benefits extend to people who aren't athletes, too. That Dutch study of nearly 6,000 men found that those with waist circumferences above 102 cm/40 in were more likely to have a condition called Sever's disease, which causes heel pain, and to develop carpal tunnel syndrome, a painful hand and wrist condition. One study even found that 70 per cent of people with carpal tunnel syndrome were either overweight or obese.

Abs Will Help You Win

IF YOU PLAY GOLF, basketball, naked Twister or any sport that requires movement, your essential muscle group isn't your chest, biceps or legs. It's your core – the muscles in your torso and hips. Developing core strength gives you power. It fortifies the muscles around your whole midsection and trains them to provide the right amount of support when you need it. So if you're weak off the tee, strong abs will improve your distance. But if you also play stop-and-start sports like tennis or basketball, abs can improve your game tremendously. Though speed is often the buzzword TV analysts like to use to differentiate between the elite and reserve-squad players, athletic success isn't really about speed. It's really about accelerating and decelerating. How fast can you go from a stopped position at point A to stopping at point B? Your legs don't control that; your abs do. When researchers studied what muscles were the first to engage in these types of sports movements, they found that the abs fired first. The stronger they are, the faster you'll get to the ball.

• • •

These are all great reasons to pursue the Abs Diet. But the best reason is this: the programme is an easy, sacrifice-free plan that will let you eat the foods you want and keep you looking and feeling better day after day. It's designed to help you lose weight in the easiest possible ways: by recalibrating your body's internal fat-burning furnace, by focusing on the foods that trigger your body to start shedding flab, and by rebuilding you into a lean, mean, fat-burning machine.

ABS DIET HEALTH BULLETIN

WHAT THE HECK IS . . . HIGH BLOOD PRESSURE?

You know high blood pressure is bad, but you probably have a little trouble getting your head around the whole concept of how 'blood pressure' works. 'Can't we just let a little of the blood out and lower the pressure?' you might wonder. If only it were so easy.

When most people think of blood pressure, they think in terms of a garden hose: too much pressure and the hose bursts, unless you open the valve. But that model is too simple. It helps instead to think of your circulatory system as more like the Grand Union Canal – a series of locks and gates that help move blood around to where it's needed. See, gravity works on your blood just like it works on the rest of your body: it wants to pull everything downwards. So imagine yourself hopping out of bed tomorrow morning and standing up. Gravity wants to take all that blood that's distributed throughout your body and pull it down into your feet. You, on the other hand, would like that blood to pump to your brain, where it can help you figure out where the hell your keys are.

On cue, arteries in the lower body constrict while the heart dramatically increases output. The instant result: blood pressure rises, and blood flows to the brain. Ahh, there they are – in the dog's water dish, right where you left them.

It's an ingenious system, but one that's incredibly easy to throw out of whack. When you pack on extra padding around your gut, your heart pumps harder to force blood into all that new fatty tissue. When you nosh on crisps and other high-sodium foods, your body retains water in order to dilute the excess salt, increasing overall blood volume. When you line your arteries with plaque from too many fatty meals, pressure increases as the same amount of blood has to squeeze through newly narrowed vessels. When you let the pressures of the day haunt you into the night, your brain pumps out stress hormones that keep your body in a perpetual state of fight-or-flight anxiousness, also forcing your heart to pump harder. High-salt, high-fat diets and an excess of stress all combine to create a dangerous situation.

Much to the dismay of Quentin Tarantino fans, letting out some blood won't relieve the pressure. Your heart is still pumping, and your blood vessels are still dilating and contracting to make sure the blood goes where it's needed. When the pressure remains high for years on end, thin-walled vessels in the brain can burst under extreme pressure; brain cells die as a result in what's known as a haemorrhagic stroke. Or hypertension can cause plaque build-up in one of the brain's arteries, eventually cutting off bloodflow. (High blood pressure damages smooth artery walls, creating anchor points for plaque to latch onto.) Kidney failure or a heart attack can also follow from dangerous plaque accumulations.

Then there's the plain old wear and tear that high blood pressure causes on your ticker. Over time, the extra work brought on by high blood pressure causes the walls of the heart to stiffen and thicken. The heart becomes a less efficient pump, unable to push out as much blood as it takes in. Blood backs up, the heart gives out, and the coroner scribbles 'congestive heart failure' on your chart.

Ideally, your blood pressure should be 120/80 or lower. What do those numbers mean? The top number, called the *systolic* pressure, is the pressure generated when the heart beats. The bottom number is the *diastolic* pressure, the pressure on your blood vessels when the heart is resting between beats. Higher readings are broken down into three categories:

▶ **Prehypertensive: 120–139 systolic/80–89 diastolic.** Prehypertensives should start worrying now about their blood pressure, concentrating on diet and exercise tips like those found in the Abs Diet. You may not see the flashing lights in your mirror right now, but your radar detector just went off. Time to slow down.

▶ **Stage I hypertensive: 140–159 systolic/90–99 diastolic.** For people who fall in this range, drug therapy is usually recommended in addition to lifestyle changes. Your risk of heart attack or stroke is elevated, and you need to be under a doctor's care.

▶ **Stage II hypertensive: 160 or greater systolic/100 or greater diastolic.** Advanced drug therapy is often a must for people at this level, who face a serious risk of being maimed or killed by their condition.

So, two questions. Do you know what your blood pressure is? If not, are you freaked out enough by now to start taking care of it? Fortunately, the Abs Diet Powerfoods can help by cutting down on the bad fats in your diet and increasing the good ones – and by slashing away some of that extra weight. So can the Abs Diet Workout, as well as a few stress-reduction techniques. (To find out how you can help manage your stress level, see 'How Stress Makes You Fat' on page 172.) In the meantime, try attacking the problem with some of these simple tips.

Make it a V8. A can of V8 (330 ml/11 fl oz) contains nearly 800 milligrams (mg) of potassium. In a study published in the *Journal of Human Hypertension*, researchers found that prehypertensive patients who added

(continued)

ABS DIET HEALTH BULLETIN

WHAT THE HECK IS . . . HIGH BLOOD PRESSURE?
(CONT.)

more potassium to their diets lowered their systolic pressure by 2.5 points and their diastolic by 1.6 points. Potassium helps sweep excess sodium from the circulatory system, causing the blood vessels to dilate. What makes V8 better than a banana (another good source of potassium)? V8 also contains lycopene and lutein, two phytochemicals that have their own blood pressure-lowering properties.

Cut out the cold cuts. One slice of ham contains 240 milligrams of sodium, more salt than you'll find on the outside of two pretzel rods. The point: lose the lunchmeat, and lower your blood pressure. A recent study found that prehypertensive people who reduced their daily sodium consumption from 3,300 to 1,500 milligrams knocked nearly 6 points off their systolic blood pressure and close to 3 off their diastolic. If you want to have your sandwich and eat it, too, at least switch to a low-sodium brand of meat – ham, turkey, roast beef – and leave the pickle on your plate (833 milligrams of sodium). Another rule of thumb: if a food comes canned or jarred, it's probably a salt mine.

Go two rounds and out. Make the second drink of the night your last call for alcohol. In a landmark study published in the *New England Journal of Medicine*, researchers found that one or two drinks a day actually decreased blood pressure slightly. Three drinks or more a day, however, elevated blood pressure by an average of 10 points systolic and 4 diastolic. The type of alcohol doesn't matter. Heck, order a screwdriver: orange juice is one of the best sources of blood pressure-lowering potassium.

Drink more tea. An American study found that men who drank two cups of tea a day were 25 per cent less likely to die of heart disease than men who rarely touched the stuff. The reason: flavonoids in the tea not only improve blood vessels' ability to relax but also thin the blood, reducing clotting.

Top your toast. Blackcurrant jelly is a good source of quercetin, an antioxidant that Finnish researchers believe may improve heart health by preventing the build-up of the free radicals that can damage arterial walls and allow plaque to penetrate.

Grab a Granny (Smith). Men who frequently eat apples have a 20 per cent lower risk of developing heart disease than men who eat apples less often.

Eat fresh berries. Raspberries, strawberries and blueberries are all loaded with salicylic acid – the same heart disease fighter found in aspirin.

Order the tuna. Omega-3 fats in tuna and other fish as well as flaxseed help strengthen heart muscle, lower blood pressure, prevent clotting and reduce levels of potentially deadly inflammation in the body.

Squeeze a grapefruit. One grapefruit a day can reduce arterial narrowing by 46 per cent, lower your bad cholesterol level by more than 10 per cent and help reduce your blood pressure by more than 5 points.

Feast on potassium. Slice a banana (487 milligrams) on your cereal, and bake a sweet potato (694 mg) or cook up some spinach for dinner (170 g/6 oz cooked spinach, 792 mg). All are loaded with potassium. Studies show that not getting at least 2,000 milligrams of potassium daily can set you up for high blood pressure. Other good sources of potassium include raisins (145 g/5 oz, 1,086 mg), tomatoes (240 ml/8 fl oz passata/sieved tomatoes, 811 mg), beans (170 g/6 oz canned red kidney beans, 402 mg) and papayas (one has 781 mg of the mineral).

Buy calcium-fortified orange juice. Increasing the calcium in your diet can lower your blood pressure. You'll derive a benefit from the vitamin C as well. According to research in England, people with the most vitamin C in their bloodstreams are 40 per cent less likely to die of heart disease.

Snack on pumpkin seeds. Thirty grams/1 oz of seeds contains 151 mg of magnesium, more than a third of your recommended daily intake. Magnesium deficiencies have been linked to most risk factors for heart disease, including high blood pressure, elevated cholesterol levels, and increased build-up of plaque in the arteries. Other great sources: halibut (200 g/7 oz, 187 mg), brown rice (200 g/7 oz cooked rice, 86 mg), chickpeas (170 g/6 oz, 82 mg), cashews (30 g/1 oz, 74 mg) and artichokes (one gives you 72 mg).

Change your oil. Researchers in India found that men who replaced the corn and vegetable oils in their kitchens with monounsaturated fats (olive oil or, in this case, sesame seed oil) lowered their blood pressure by more than 30 points in just 60 days without making any other changes in their diets.

Cut down on mindless sweet snacking. A compound in liquorice root has been shown to spike blood pressure – especially in men who eat a lot of black liquorice. Fruit-flavored liquorice, however, doesn't contain the compound.

THE ABS DIET START-UP KIT

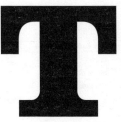**HIS SIMPLE SHOPPING LIST WILL** give you everything you need to dive right in to the Abs Diet and the Abs Diet Workout.

Buy Once

Blender	Ground flaxseed	Multivitamins, such as Wellman, plus chromium supplement

Basic Shopping List – The ABS DIET POWER 12 and Related Foods

Almonds, slivered or whole

Beans of choice

Spinach, fresh or frozen

Dairy (skimmed milk, fat-free or low-fat yogurt)

Instant hot oat cereal (unsweetened, unflavoured)

Eggs

Turkey

Peanut butter, natural (no added sugar)

Olive oil

Wholegrain breads and cereals

Extra-protein (whey) powder

Raspberries and other berries (fresh and frozen)

Plus:

Canned tuna

Chicken breast

Cooking oil spray

Grapefruit, oranges or other fruit of choice

Green vegetables of choice

Lean fish of choice

Lean minced beef

Long-grain brown rice

Whole-wheat pasta

Shopping List – Ingredients for Recipes
(see recipes for individual amounts)

Back bacon

Balsamic vinegar

Bananas

Black beans

Breadcrumbs

Brown rice

Carrots

Chicken stock, fresh or frozen

Celery

Chickpeas

Chilli and garlic sauce

Chilli powder

Curry powder

Dried chilli mix

Flour

Fresh red and green chillies

Fresh ginger

Garlic

Green and red peppers

Guacamole

Haricot beans

Honey

Honeydew melon

Italian seasoning

Ketchup

Lean sirloin steak

Lean sliced roast beef

Lemons

Limes

Low-fat Italian salad dressing

Mayonnaise (light or fat-free)

Mushrooms

Onions

Onion soup mix

Orange juice

Orange juice concentrate, frozen

Paprika

Parmesan cheese

Pasta sauce

Reduced-fat cheese (Cheddar, cream, mozzarella, string cheese sticks)

Raisins

Romaine (Cos) lettuce

Salmon fillets

Salsa

Sweetcorn, canned or frozen

Tabasco sauce

Tomatoes, fresh and canned

Tomato sauce

Tortillas

Trans fat-free spread

Turkey bacon

Turkey sausages

Wholemeal muffins

Wholewheat pittas

Worcestershire sauce

For At-Home Exercise
(if you belong to a gym, they should have all necessary equipment)

Exercise mat (optional)

Flat bench (optional, but recommended)

One or two pairs of medium-weight dumbbells (2.25 to 12 kg/ 5 to 26 lb for someone with some experience lifting weights; lighter for beginners)

Running shoes

Swiss ball (optional, but recommended)

Chapter 2

WHY THE ABS DIET? AND WHY NOW?

Shocking New Scientific Breakthroughs in Nutrition

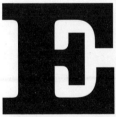**ARLIER IN THIS BOOK, I OUTLINED** half a dozen ways the Abs Diet will improve your life. And I told you about the unique and scientifically proven promise of the Abs Diet, how it can strip off up to 9 kg/20 lb of fat in 6 weeks – starting with your stomach. But the next steps are up to you.

If you're simply not interested in improving your life – if the idea of becoming a slimmer, fitter, healthier, pain-free, more successful, more sexually vital person doesn't appeal to you – then close this book right now, and return it. (After you wipe off the chip grease stains, of course.) If you're not interested in achieving the greatest possible results with the least possible effort, this book is not for you.

But if you do want to make a change – one you can see, one you can feel, one that will last a lifetime – then this book is for you. The only one for you.

The Abs Diet is a simple plan built around 12 nutrient-packed foods that, when moved to the head of your dietary table, will give you all the vitamins, minerals and fibre you need for optimum health while triggering muscle growth and firing up your body's natural fat burners. I'll tell you more about these foods in a later chapter, but here's a quick overview. (Tell me this isn't a meal plan you can stick to!)

Almonds and other nuts

Beans and pulses

Spinach and other green vegetables

Dairy (skimmed milk, fat-free or low-fat yogurt and cheese)

Instant hot oat cereal (unsweetened, unflavoured)

Eggs

Turkey and other lean meats

Peanut butter

Olive oil

Wholegrain breads and cereals

Extra-protein (whey) powder

Raspberries and other berries

12!

I've chosen these foods both for their nutritional content and for their simplicity. See, every day, new diet books and weight-loss advice shuffle across my desk. (In fact, if you plug 'diet' in to

Amazon.com's search engine, you'll turn up more than 80,000 titles.) Some of these diet schemes are a little wacky: grapefruit diets, cabbage soup diets, cottage cheese diets. Some of them sound good – low-fat diets, low-carb diets, low-salt diets. But most of them have one thing in common: they are actually designed to make you fail in the long run.

That's because even the diet plans that are based on sound principles sometimes fail to acknowledge the realities of life – that you're too busy to whip up intricate meals like mango-flavoured prawn kebabs. That you enjoy food too much to swear off pasta and potatoes all the time. That eating is supposed to be a pleasure, not a chore. That's why I based the Abs Diet on common foods that are easy to prepare and enjoy. The way I see it, most other diet plans are too complicated and invite failure in three major ways.

1. They reduce calories too severely. With a strict – or drastic – calorie reduction, you may lose weight at first, but you're left hungry. When you're hungry, you've increased the chances that you'll gorge at some point during the day. When you gorge, you feel as if you failed, then feel guilty for failing, then drop off the plan and resume your cold-pizza-for-breakfast habits. With the Abs Diet, however, you'll never go hungry – in fact, you'll find yourself eating much more often than you do now: six times a day!

2. They restrict too many foods. It would be easy to build a plan that didn't include burgers, pizza or beer. But if I did that, you'd ditch the plan on the first afternoon of the football season. Even though changing your eating habits is a fundamental part of this programme, I think there's a greater chance you'll stick to the plan if you don't have to give up everything you like. It's normal to have steaks with clients, to have hot dogs at a barbecue, to have a pint of beer after work. If you deprive yourself of every food that tastes good, there's not much incentive for even the most motivated person to stick to the plan for longer than a few weeks. The Abs Diet is about eating the foods you enjoy – and indulging yourself when need be.

3. They don't take into account lifestyle. If we all had a chef to prepare our meals – or even more than a few minutes to do it ourselves – losing weight would be much simpler. But when was the last time you had 2 hours to prepare a meal? We're all busy. We eat in restaurants. We order in. We hit drive-throughs. We wish we had time to tally fat-gram totals, weigh each portion of food or prepare elaborate good-for-you dishes. But the reality is that most of us won't, no matter how much weight we need to lose. We have commitments to jobs and families, and we spend so much time doing everything from commuting to fixing our home that a mango-prawn masterpiece is what slips down on our priority list. The Abs Diet is what you need: a low-maintenance programme, with low-maintenance foods and even lower-maintenance recipes.

Let's take a look at a handful of today's most popular diets, and I'll show you why many of them are designed to offer short-term weight loss and long-term weight gain.

The Atkins Diet: Limiting Food, Limiting Nutrition

THE ATKINS DIET eliminates practically all carbohydrates for the first part of the plan, leaving you with only foods that contain protein and fat: no bread, no pasta, no fruit, no vegetables, no juice – no fun. The Atkins diet, no question, helps people lose weight. I've seen men lose up to 13.6 kg/30 lb on Atkins – all of them feasting on steak, cheese and bacon while doing so, and I've seen the studies that support the plan's effectiveness in helping people lose weight, at least in the short term. Emphasizing protein is smart, but eliminating many other foods that are important to maintaining good health isn't. But here's my real issue with this kind of diet, one that often gets overlooked in the whole no carbohydrate debate. I could restrict you to any couple of foods – let's say chips, ice cream and burgers. Go on a diet eating just those things, and chances are that you'd lose weight – because you simply can't force yourself to eat the same stuff over and over again. By restricting the foods you eat to only a handful of them, you'll automatically lose weight because you've dramatically reduced your total calories. But you've also dramatically reduced your intake of vitamins, minerals and fibre, while upping your intake of artery-clogging saturated fats. Even more important, you just couldn't stay on such a diet long-term, no matter how much you liked it, because your lifestyle (and taste buds) demand a more flexible, more enjoyable eating plan – and because your body is programmed to crave fruits and grains and juices just as much as it craves burgers and chips.

Well, as crazy as it sounds, that super-restrictive, low-nutrient diet is exactly what you get with Atkins. You eat a limited number of foods – the vast majority containing protein and saturated fat. You'll lose weight because you've eliminated carbohydrates, but you've also put yourself at risk of a number of health problems. For one, the foods on Atkins have high amounts of saturated fats, and there's overwhelming evidence that societies with diets high in saturated fats face a greater prevalence of heart disease. Secondly, by eliminating most carbohydrates from your diet, you're eliminating some important nutrients, like vitamin B and fibre and phytonutrients that help your immune system. Worst of all, even though Atkins does introduce carbohydrates later in the plan, few people can stick to the limited number of foods that Atkins allows. So that short-term weight loss leads to long-term weight gain and, potentially, long-term health problems.

Weight Watchers: Too Much Maths, Too Little Food

WEIGHT WATCHERS – a popular point-tallying system that enforces portion control by having you log the amount of food you eat every day – works for many people. Those who overeat can benefit by tracking what they consume and being conscious of reducing calories. But this programme has its flaws. First, I don't know many people who have the time or long-term discipline to measure foods and count calories on a daily basis. Secondly, Weight Watchers doesn't guarantee nutritional balance. You could count your points so that you eat nothing but junk if you skimped during other parts of the day. In theory, you could eat your day's worth of points at one or two meals – and that would slow down your metabolism and might actually make you gain weight. Calorie counting, as I'll explain, is only one component of a successful weight-control programme. Thirdly, and most important, a lot of people don't like the support group atmosphere of Weight Watchers.

The Zone: A Too-Delicate Balancing Act

THE ZONE DIET, by Dr Barry Sears, involves balancing the kinds of food that you eat with the goal of putting you 'in the Zone'. The basic premise is that at every meal you should have carbs, protein and a little bit of monounsaturated fat in the precise ratio that Sears recommends. Carbs are divided into desirable carbs, such as vegetables and some fruit, and undesirable carbs, such as bread, juice, beer and cakes. Proteins and fats are divided similarly. This gives you freedom to eat what you want, but when choosing undesirable foods, you must eat less of them and they must be accompanied by other foods. For example, you can indulge in 'bad' carbs, but only in moderation, and you must accompany them with protein and some fat. So if you're planning to have a beer, plan on a helping of cottage cheese and a few olives to balance it out. This is why many people complain about the Zone –

some of the food combos can be out of the ordinary, and measuring how much of each group you can and should eat can be overly complicated. Sears provides formulas to determine how much of which foods you should eat based on how much you exercise and your level of body fat. This number can be converted to how many 'blocks' of each food you should have in a day. You can distribute them throughout the day but not let 5 hours pass between meals. The business of measuring, dividing and combining can get pretty complex to manage; even though the balance of food is pretty sensible, you'd have to be an air traffic controller to keep everything straight. The diet is so reliant on its central gimmick that almost no one has the time or energy to follow it for very long.

Sugar Busters: Making Sweets a Sin

THE SUGAR BUSTERS DIET philosophy centres around eliminating foods high in sugar as well as foods that spike your blood sugar and make you hungry (like some carbohydrates such as pasta, sweetcorn, beer and potatoes). The benefit, proponents say, is that if you follow the plan, you'll be able to enjoy steak, eggs and cheese – and still lose weight. But simply eating less sugar won't help you lose weight. Without nutritional balance, you can still consume a lot of high-calorie foods that are low in sugar and end up gaining weight. And as with other diets, you've done nothing to change the way your body processes foods to achieve the highest calorie burn that you can.

Dr Phil: Just a Little Too Emotional

DR PHIL MCGRAW, the pop psychologist who made it big as the tough-love guru on Oprah's talk show, has a diet programme that's hugely popular in the States; the main emphasis is on stripping food of its emotional power. McGraw's book, *The Ultimate Weight Solution: The 7 Keys to Weight Loss Freedom*, stresses the notion that we've allowed food to have too much power in our lives and that, in order to quit binge eating, we need to (a) limit our access to junk food, (b) select foods that take a long time to prepare and chew so that it's harder for us to eat, and (c) stop eating to satisfy cravings and feelings of stress. Sounds good, except that in today's world, Antarctica is about the only place that doesn't have convenient access to junk food. I agree that we should stop eating to satisfy cravings and stress, and I applaud Dr Phil for recognizing the psychological aspects of our eating habits. What the Abs Diet does is show you how to eat to prevent cravings and stress. The Abs Diet makes it easy to snack smartly throughout the day, so you'll never go hungry. It also helps you take control of your food intake, your body and your life, so you can beat back stress.

The South Beach Diet: Eating Right Is Just the Start

IN HIS FIRST BOOK, *THE SOUTH BEACH DIET*, cardiologist Dr Arthur Agatston emphasized balanced eating, relying on lean protein, good fats and good carbohydrates. As you'll see, some of South Beach's nutritional principles are similar to those of the Abs Diet. Dr Agatston focuses heavily on the role of insulin and how spikes in blood sugar make you hungry. His follow-up book *The South Beach Diet Supercharged* adds a crucial component missing from the first: exercise. It shows you how to tune up your metabolism, your body's natural fat burner. The total-body toning exercises and walking interval workouts are terrific for beginners just starting on the road to fitness, but the workouts may be a bit light for those who want to amp up their weight loss and take fitness to another level. *The Abs Diet*, on the other hand, incorporates strength-building exercises with weights, which appear to directly fight abdominal fat, according to studies by the National Institutes of Health in the US and the University of Pennsylvania. By revving up your body's fat-burning mechanism, you can take control over not only the calories coming into your body but also the calories being burned by it. Strength training can also reduce your risk of developing diabetes. Researchers at the University of Massachusetts found that men who added two total-body weight workouts a week to their regular cardio exercise had post-meal insulin levels that were 25 per cent lower after those of men who did aerobics but didn't lift weights.

• • •

As I said at the beginning of this book, most diets are about losing. The Abs Diet is about gaining. The Abs Diet is based on the notion that your body is a living, breathing, calorie-burning machine, and that by keeping your body's fat furnace constantly stoked with lots of the right foods – and this is important – at the right time, you can teach it to start burning off your belly in no time. In fact, this diet can help you burn up to 5.4 kg/12 lb of fat – from your belly first – in 2 weeks or less. And just look at what you'll gain in return.

You'll gain meals. Many of us have huge appetites. We hunger for success, we hunger for freedom and, yeah, we hunger for food. Traditional calorie- or food-restricting diets run counter to this kind of appetite. They leave us hungry, miserable and one snap away from going psycho in the snacks aisle. But not the Abs Diet. You will eat on this programme – and eat often. In fact, you'll be refuelling constantly, and with every delicious meal or snack, you'll be stoking your body's natural fat burners. Imagine that: every time you eat, you help your body lose weight and turn flab into abs.

You'll gain muscle. With the Abs Diet and the Abs Diet Workout, the more you eat, the more muscle you'll build, and the more fat you'll lose. This programme converts the food you eat into muscle. The more lean muscle mass you have, the more energy it takes to fuel it – meaning that calories go to your muscles to sustain them rather than to convert to fat. In fact, research shows that adding lean muscle mass acts as a built-in fat burner. Again, for every ½ kg/1 lb of muscle you gain, your resting metabolic rate goes up as much as 50 calories a day. The strength-training component can put several kg/lb of muscle onto your body. You won't beef up like a bodybuilder, but you will build enough muscle to shrink and tighten your gut – and, depending on your starting point, show off your abs. When you add exercise into the mix, you can think of it as a simple equation:

MORE FOOD = **MORE MUSCLE** = **LESS FLAB**

Now, consider the alternative:

LESS FOOD = **LESS MUSCLE** = **MORE FLAB**

Isn't it incredible that most diets focus on the 'less food' equation? And isn't it time we changed that? (Sure, some studies have shown that you'll live longer on a super-restrictive diet of less than 1,400 calories a day. But given how such a plan would make you feel, you probably wouldn't want to.)

You'll gain freedom. Most diets deprive you of something – whether it's carbs, fat or your manhood. (Tofu? No thanks.) In this plan, you will not feel deprived. You'll stay full. You'll eat crunchy food. You'll eat sweet food. You'll eat protein, carbs and fat. In fact, there's even one meal during the week when you can eat anything

---

ABS DIET SUCCESS STORY

'I WENT FROM BRANDO TO RAMBO!'

Name: Bill Stanton

Age: 40

Height: 1.72 m/5'8"

Starting weight: 99.8 kg/15 st 10 lb

Six weeks later: 86.2 kg/13 st 8 lb

Bill Stanton, a security consultant, had been pumping iron since he was 15. But even with his rigorous weight training, he kept getting fatter: by the time he reached 40, he had ballooned to 99.8 kg/15 st 10 lb on his 1.72-m/5 ft 8-in frame. Why? Because his diet and exercise routine consisted of doing bench presses and squats and then finishing the night with chicken wings and booze.

'My trousers were fitting me like a tourniquet, and it was like I was in a bad marriage – I was living comfortably uncomfortable,' Stanton says. 'The Abs Diet challenged me to get on the programme, step up to the plate, and step away from the plate.'

you want. Anything. During the bulk of the week, you'll focus on foods that will charge your metabolism and control your temptations, but you'll also have the freedom and flexibility to stray just enough to keep you satisfied without ruining all the work you've already put in.

You'll gain time. On some diets, it seems like it would take less time to organize a hunting party and stalk a woolly mammoth than it would take to plan and cook the recipes they tout. On this diet, all of the meals and recipes are low-maintenance. For planning purposes, all I want you to do is take this programme 2 days at a time. Since mindless noshing is the number one diet buster, your best defence is to plot out a simple strategy for how and what you're going to eat each day. Every night, take 5 minutes to sketch out what and when you'll eat the next day, and you'll have deflated temptation and gained control. After reading the principles, you'll see that the Abs Diet establishes a new paradigm for weight control. Simply:

MORE FOOD = MORE MUSCLE = LESS FLAB

After following the Abs Diet for 6 weeks, Stanton lost 13.6 kg/30 lb – and has cut his body fat from 30 per cent to 15 per cent. 'I looked pregnant. I looked like a power lifter – big arms, a big chest, and a big gut. Now I look like Rambo.'

Stanton appreciated the diversity of the Abs Diet meals and the plan's total-body approach to working out, though he admits that eating six times a day took some getting used to. 'What I had to do was learn to eat to live, not live to eat,' he says. And then, he says, everything just rolled from there. Once his mental approach changed – being committed to the plan, limiting the number of times he partied at night, and eliminating late-night meals – he was able to turn everything around. 'You wake up attacking the day rather than waiting for the day to end,' he says.

Now, everything just feels better. He's always in a good mood. He walks taller. He has more energy. And now he's a model for others.

'I work out at Sports Club LA, where people are *really* focused on looking great,' he says. 'Even there, guys and girls all come up to me. One guy said, "You are kicking butt. Everybody sees that transformation. You're inspiring a lot of people."'

Stanton has changed his physique so dramatically that he's even been accused of taking steroids. 'I take that as a compliment,' he laughs.

ABS DIET HEALTH BULLETIN

WHAT THE HECK IS . . . HIGH CHOLESTEROL?

Cholesterol is a soft, waxy substance found among the lipids (fats) in the bloodstream and in all your body's cells. For all the bad press it gets, the fact is that you need cholesterol, because your body uses it to form cell membranes, create hormones and perform several other crucial maintenance operations. But a high level of cholesterol in the blood – hypercholesterolaemia – is a major risk factor for coronary heart disease, which leads to heart attack.

You get cholesterol in two ways. The body – mainly the liver – produces varying amounts, usually about 1,000 milligrams a day. But when you consume foods high in saturated fats – particularly trans fats – your body goes cholesterol crazy, pumping out more than you could ever use. (Some foods also contain cholesterol, especially egg yolks, meat, poultry, fish, seafood, and whole-milk dairy products. But the majority of it, and the stuff I want you to focus on, is made by your own body.)

Some of the excess cholesterol in your bloodstream is removed from the body through the liver. But some of it winds up exactly where you don't want it – along the walls of your arteries, where it combines with other substances to form plaque. Plaque is bad for several reasons: first, it raises blood pressure by making your heart work harder to get blood through your suddenly narrower blood vessels, which can eventually wear out your ticker. Secondly, plaque can break off its little perch and tumble through your bloodstream, eventually forming a clot that can lead to stroke, paralysis, death and other annoyances.

Inside your body, a war is raging right now between two factions of specialized sherpas called lipoproteins that are moving cholesterol around your insides according to their own specialized agendas. There are several kinds, but the ones to focus on are the Jekyll and Hyde of health, HDL (high-density or 'helpful' lipoprotein) and LDL (low-density or 'lazy' lipo-protein) cholesterol.

The good guy: HDL cholesterol. About a quarter to one-third of blood cholesterol is carried by helpful HDL. HDL wants to help you out by picking up cholesterol and getting it the hell out of your bloodstream by carrying it back to the liver, where it's passed from the body. That's good. Some experts believe that HDL removes excess cholesterol from plaques and thus slows their growth. That's really good. A high HDL level seems to protect against heart attack. The opposite is also true: a low HDL level (less than 1 millimole per litre (mmol/L) indicates a greater risk. A low HDL cholesterol level may also raise stroke risk.

The bad guy: LDL cholesterol. Lazy LDL has no interest at all in helping you out. LDL just wants to stick cholesterol in the most convenient place it can find, meaning your arteries. LDL doesn't care that too much cholesterol lining your arteries causes a build-up of plaque, a condition known as atherosclerosis. A high level of LDL cholesterol (3.0 mmol/L) reflects an increased risk of heart disease. Lower levels of LDL cholesterol reflect a lower risk of heart disease.

Simply put, HDL is trying to come to your aid, but LDL is just sitting there, laughing at you. If you want to give HDL a hand, start stocking up on the Abs Diet Powerfoods, and follow the guidelines of the Abs Diet Workout. Here are some more quick ideas on beating the bad guy for good.

Butt out. Tobacco smoking is one of the six major risk factors of heart disease that you can change or treat. Smoking lowers HDL (good) cholesterol levels.

Drink up. In some studies, moderate use of alcohol is linked with higher HDL (good) cholesterol levels. But take it easy there, Dino. People who consume moderate amounts of alcohol (an average of one to two drinks per day for men and one drink per day for women) have a lower risk of heart disease, but increased consumption of alcohol can bring other health dangers, such as alcoholism, high blood pressure, obesity and cancer.

Johnny B good. A B vitamin called niacin reduces LDL (bad) cholesterol at the same time it raises beneficial HDL. In fact, niacin can be more effective at treating these things than popular cholesterol-busting drugs, which tend to act more generally on total cholesterol and gross LDL. (Be careful, though. While the niacin you get from foods and over-the-counter vitamins is fine, super-high doses of niacin can have serious side effects and should be taken only under a doctor's supervision.)

Tea it up. Three recent studies confirm that drinking green tea can help lower your cholesterol level and reduce your risk of developing cancer. In a 12-week trial of 240 men and women, researchers at Vanderbilt University found that drinking the equivalent of 7 cups of green tea a day can help lower LDL (bad) cholesterol levels by 16 per cent. Seven cups a day is a lot of tea, but even 1 or 2 cups a day could have a beneficial impact.

Meanwhile, researchers at the University of Rochester recently determined that green tea extract can help prevent the growth of cancer cells, and Medical College of Ohio researchers found that a compound called EGCG in green tea may help slow or stop the progression of bladder cancer.

Go for the grapefruit. If you want to make one simple dietary change for better health, the best thing you can do is eat a single white or ruby grapefruit

(continued)

ABS DIET HEALTH BULLETIN

WHAT THE HECK IS . . . HIGH CHOLESTEROL?
(CONT.)

every day. Grapefruit is gaining ground as a powerfood. New research shows that it can fight heart disease and cancer, trigger your body to lose weight, and even help you get a better night's sleep. A grapefruit a day can lower your total cholesterol and LDL (bad) cholesterol levels by 8 and 11 per cent, respectively.

Cram in the cranberry. Researchers at the University of Scranton in Pennsylvania found that men who drank three glasses of cranberry juice daily raised their HDL (good) cholesterol levels by 10 per cent, which in turn lowered their risk of heart disease by 40 per cent. Plant compounds called polyphenols are believed to be responsible for the effect. (*Note:* Cranberry juice often comes diluted, so make sure the label says that it contains at least 27 per cent cranberry juice.)

Spread some on. Instead of butter or margarine, try Benecol spread. It contains stanol ester, a plant substance that inhibits cholesterol absorption. A study at the Mayo Clinic found that people eating 4½ tablespoons of Benecol daily lowered their LDL (bad) cholesterol by 14 per cent in 8 weeks. When they stopped using it, their LDL returned to previous levels. Benecol can also be used for cooking.

Gain with grains and beans. Researchers at St Michael's Hospital in Toronto had people add several servings of foods like whole grains, nuts and beans to their diets each day. One month later, the test subjects' LDL (bad) cholesterol levels were nearly 30 per cent lower than when the trial began. In another study, this one at Tulane University, researchers found that people who ate four or more servings a week had a 22 per cent lower risk of developing heart disease (and 75 per cent fewer camping companions) than less-than-once-a-week bean eaters.

Don't let your tank hit empty. A study in the *British Medical Journal* found that people who eat six or more small meals a day have 5 per cent lower cholesterol levels than those who eat one or two large meals. That's enough to shrink your risk of heart disease by 10 to 20 per cent.

Refrain from fries. In a study published in the *New England Journal of Medicine*, the exercise and nutritional habits of 80,000 women were recorded for 14 years. The researchers found that the most important correlate of heart disease was the women's dietary intake of foods containing trans fatty acids, mutated forms of fat that lower HDL (good) and increase LDL (bad) cholesterol. Some of the worst offenders are french fries.

Sow your oats. In a University of Connecticut study, men with high cholesterol who ate oat bran cookies daily for 8 weeks lowered their levels of LDL cholesterol by more than 20 per cent. So eat more oat bran fibre, such as porridge or Cheerios. A study in the *American Journal of Clinical Nutrition* reports that two servings of wholegrain cereal (Cheerios count) a day can reduce a man's risk of dying of heart disease by nearly 20 per cent.

Rise and dine. In a study of 3,900 people, Harvard researchers found that men who ate breakfast every day were 44 per cent less likely to be overweight and 41 per cent less likely to develop insulin resistance, both risk factors for heart disease.

Fortify with folic acid. A study published in the *British Medical Journal* found that people who consume the recommended amount of folic acid each day have a 16 per cent lower risk of heart disease than those whose diets are lacking in this B vitamin. Good sources of folic acid include asparagus, broccoli and fortified cereal.

Order a salad. Leafy greens and egg yolks are both good sources of lutein, a phytochemical that carries heart disease-fighting antioxidants to your cells and tissues.

Be a sponge. Loma Linda University researchers found that drinking five or more 240-ml/8-fl oz glasses of water a day could help lower your risk of heart disease by up to 60 per cent – exactly the same drop you get from stopping smoking, lowering your LDL (bad) cholesterol numbers, exercising or losing a little weight.

Give yourself bad breath. In addition to lowering cholesterol and helping to fight off infection, eating garlic may help limit damage to your heart after a heart attack or heart surgery. Researchers in India found that animals that were fed garlic regularly had more heart-protecting antioxidants in their blood than animals that weren't.

Crank up the chromium. According to new research from Harvard, men with low levels of chromium in their systems are significantly more likely to develop heart problems. You need between 200 and 400 micrograms of chromium per day – more than you're likely to get from your regular diet. Look for a supplement labelled chromium picolinate; it's the most easily absorbed by the body.

Snack on nuts. Harvard researchers found that men who replaced 127 calories of carbohydrates – that's one small packet of crisps – with 30 g/1 oz of nuts decreased their risk of heart disease by 30 per cent.

Chapter 3

BURN FAT DAY AND NIGHT
How Metabolism Shapes Your Body –
And How You Can Change Yours

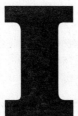N CHAPTER 2, I DISCUSSED HOW MOST popular diets are designed to offer only short-term weight loss, and how following these programmes sets you up not only to regain the weight you initially shed but to actually gain even more fat in the long run. Most diets, in fact, are not long-term fat-loss plans but long-term muscle-loss plans. The Abs Diet is different: it's a programme that helps you rev up your body's natural fat burners and keep them revved up for life.

As harmful as most diet crazes may be, diets alone aren't to blame for the West's obesity epidemic. In fact, there's plenty of blame to go around: fast food, stress, sedentary lifestyles, supersizing, all-you-can-eat buffets, the demise of physical education classes, free refills, sofas, cinema popcorn, you name it. But in the battle of weight control, these are the easy targets. Instead, I'd argue, one of the reasons we keep getting fatter is that we put our faith in two things that are supposed to help us lose weight. These weight loss 'double agents' reap praise for their contributions to good health, but they've also done their part in skewing the way we think about weight loss. The two culprits I blame for our obesity epidemic? Nutritional labels and exercise machines.

The Case against Calorie Counting

Before you bust a button, hear me out. Labels and machines both have their appropriate uses (the former for the simple knowledge of the vitamins, minerals and ingredients in your food, the latter for getting people off their bottoms and exercising). My beef with labels and machines is not what they do *per se* but the myth they perpetuate. Through their function, they feed into a way of thinking about weight loss that actually makes it harder to control weight. They've turned us into a community of heavies who worship at the altar of one seemingly omnipotent number: the calorie.

With every food you eat and with every workout you finish, you look at how many calories come in and how many calories go out. It's the turnstile theory of weight loss: if you exercise away more than you take in, then you'll lose weight. Experts tell us that ½ kg/1 lb of fat contains roughly 3,500 calories, so if you simply delete 500 calories from your daily meals, increase your daily exercise by 500 calories, or some combination thereof, you'll lose ½ kg/1 lb of fat a week. That sounds great in theory, but in real life, the whole concept of calorie management is more likely to make you lose heart than lose weight. You hump it on the stairclimber for 30 minutes and sweat like you were in a sauna. When you see the final readout – 'Workout Completed: 300 Calories Burned!' – you feel like you've just chipped away at your belly and got closer to your goal. That is, until you reach for a midnight snack and see that a serving and a half of Sultana Bran also equals 300 calories. What took 30 minutes to burn takes 30 seconds to polish off. It's a psychological diet killer.

Of course, there's nothing wrong with using nutritional labels to track what you eat or as a deterrent to stay away from high-calorie foods in the first place. And it can be helpful to use machine readouts to gauge the intensity of your exercise. But you will derail your weight-loss efforts if you keep focusing on the number of calories you take in during meals and the number of calories you burn off during exercise. You need to focus, rather, on what is happening inside your body during the rest of your day – when you're working, sleeping, making love or just sitting still right now reading this book. Right this very instant, your body is either gaining fat or losing fat. The Abs Diet will train your body to lose fat while you're sitting still, because the Abs Diet focuses on something other diet plans miss: your metabolism.

What Is 'Metabolism'?

Metabolism is the rate at which your body burns its way through calories just to keep itself alive – to keep your heart beating, your lungs breathing, your blood pumping and your mind fantasizing about the Caribbean while crunching year-end accounting figures. Your body is burning calories all the time, even while you're reading this sentence. The average woman burns about 10 calories per ½ kg/1 lb of body weight every day; the average man, 11 calories per ½ kg/1 lb.

There are three main types of calorie burn that happen throughout your day. Understand how they work, and you'll understand exactly why the Abs Diet is going to turn your body into a fat-burning machine.

Calorie burn 1: the thermic effect of eating. Between 10 and 30 per cent of the calories you burn each day get burned by the simple act of digesting your food. Now that's pretty cool – it means that satisfying your food cravings actually makes you burn away calories. But not all foods are created equal: your body uses more calories to digest protein (about 25 calories burned for every 100 calories consumed) than it does to digest fats and

ABS DIET SUCCESS STORY

'I NOW HAVE A BELLY I CAN BARE'

Name: Jessica Guff

Age: 43

Height: 1.63 m/5'4"

Starting weight: 60 kg/9st 4lb

Six weeks later: 54.5 kg/8 st 8 lb

Jessica Guff doesn't believe in stepping on the scales. See, numbers don't give a total health picture, Guff says. What really matters is how you view yourself – not to mention how others view you, too. Take the time she was walking into a client's office. The people there hadn't seen her for a couple of weeks, and one employee said to another, 'Who's that skinny woman over there?'

'It's Jessica,' the other employee told her. 'She's on this thing called the Abs Diet.'

That exchange took place just 2 weeks after Guff started the Abs Diet – and she felt the effects immediately. Guff, who runs marathons, has always been in good shape. But the effect of having two kids had taken its toll on her tummy. 'I was in pretty good shape, except for my stomach,' she says. 'But since going on the plan, I really noticed a difference. I could probably crunch walnuts with my abs.'

carbohydrates (10 to 15 calories burned for every 100 calories consumed). That's why the Abs Diet concentrates on lean, healthy proteins. Eat more of them, in a sensible way, and you'll burn more calories.

Calorie burn 2: exercise and movement. Another 10 to 15 per cent of your calorie burn comes from moving your muscles, whether you're pressing weights overhead, running to catch the bus, or just twiddling your thumbs. Simply turning the pages of this book will burn calories.

The key for Guff was changing the way she approached eating. Sacrificing her own eating habits to get her kids out the door and keep up with her fitness training, she'd start the day with tea – and often little else. 'I used to go out and run without eating anything, and that was really stupid,' Guff says. 'I was horrified to learn the truth – that exercising on an empty stomach causes you to burn muscle, not fat.' But the simple strategies of the Abs Diet changed all that. 'Now I'm having smoothies for breakfast, and it's made me fitter and stoked up my energy,' Guff says.

Guff says she couldn't do a programme in which she'd have to count calories or weigh food. 'What I love about the Abs Diet is the flexibility,' she says. 'All I have to remember is the catchy acronym – ABS DIET POWER – and I can remember the 12 Powerfoods.'

The results: she's leaner – and stronger. When her 25.5-kg/4-st daughter fell asleep on the sofa, Guff was the one who picked her up and carried her to bed. 'I thought, either I'm getting stronger or she's losing weight,' she says.

And she's also more confident. 'When women look at other women, they look at their boobs, their bums and their waists – especially women who've had children. Every woman who's had a child cares about having a flat stomach.'

But the true measure of her success came in the form of a pair of green satin cargo trousers. Guff says, 'They're kinda hot, but my stomach shows when I wear them. I have two kids, so I have no business flashing my midsection.' But after 2 weeks on the plan, she decided to put them to the public test.

'All these people started complimenting me. A guy I went to college with said, "Nice outfit." My husband said I looked great,' Guff says. 'I'm going out tonight and I'm wearing the trousers again.'

Calorie burn 3: basal metabolism. This one's the biggie. Your basal, or resting, metabolism refers to the calories you're burning when you're doing nothing at all. Sleeping, watching TV, sitting through yet another mind-numbing presentation on corporate profit-and-loss statements – you're burning calories all the while. In fact, between 60 and 80 per cent of your daily calories are burned up just doing nothing. That's because your body is constantly in motion: your heart is beating, your lungs are breathing and your cells are dividing, all the time, even when you sleep.

Add up the percentages and you'll see that the majority of your daily calorie burn comes from physiological functions that you don't even think about – the thermic effect of eating and your basal metabolism. While exercise is important, you need to realize that the calories you burn off during exercise aren't important. Let me repeat that: exercise is important, but the calories you burn off during exercise aren't important. That's why the exercise programme we outline in the Abs Diet is designed to alter your basal metabolism, turning your downtime into fat-burning time. And it's why the food choices we outline for you are designed to maximize the number of calories you burn simply by eating and digesting. I want you to forget about the calories you're burning during those 30 minutes in the gym and concentrate on the calories you're burning the other 23½ hours a day.

In effect, the Abs Diet is going to change your body into a fat-frying dynamo by several means.

Changing the Way You Exercise

HAVE YOU EVER seen a gym at rush hour? Everyone hovers around the treadmills, elliptical trainers and stationary bikes. Signs warn you of 20-minute maximums so that the next sweat-seeker can have his turn. It seems like everyone wants a cardiovascular, aerobic workout. The more you sweat, the more calories you burn, the more weight you lose, right? In a way, yes, the headphone-and-Lycra set is right. Cardiovascular exercise – steady-state endurance exercises, like running, biking and swimming – burns a lot of calories. In fact, it often burns more than other forms of exercise like strength training or trendier workouts like yoga or Pilates. But when it comes to weight control, aerobic exercise is more overrated than the autumn TV lineup. Why? For one reason: aerobic exercise builds little (if any) muscle – and muscle is the key component of a speedy metabolism. Muscle eats fat; again, add ½ kg/1 lb of muscle, and your body burns up to an additional 50 calories a day just to keep that muscle alive. Add 2.75 kg/6 lb of muscle, and suddenly you're burning up to 300 more calories each day just by sitting still.

Here's the problem with low-intensity aerobic exercise. Just like a car can't run without fuel or a kite can't fly without wind, a body can't function without food. It's the fuel that helps you run, lift and have the legs to make love all night long. Generally, during exercise, your body calls upon glycogen (the stored form of carbohydrate in muscles and the liver), fat and, in some cases, protein. When you're doing low-intensity aerobic exercise like jogging, your body primarily uses fat and glycogen (carbohydrates) for fuel. When it continues at longer periods (20 minutes or more), your body drifts into depletion: you exhaust your first-tier energy sources (your glycogen stores), and your body hunts around for the easiest source of energy it can find – protein. Your body actually begins to eat up muscle tissue, converting the protein stored in your muscles into energy you need to keep going. Once your body reaches that plateau, it burns up 5 to 6 grams of protein for every 30 minutes of ongoing exercise. (That's roughly the amount of protein you'll find in a hard-boiled egg.) By burning protein, you're not only missing an opportunity to burn fat but also losing all-important and powerful muscle. So aerobic exercise actually decreases muscle mass. Decreased muscle mass ultimately slows down your metabolism, making it easier for you to gain weight.

Now here's an even more shocking fact: when early studies compared cardiovascular exercise to weight training, researchers learned that those who engaged in aerobic activities burned more calories during exercise than those who tossed around iron. You'd assume, then, that aerobic exercise was the way to go. But that's not the end of the story.

It turns out that while weight lifters didn't burn as many calories during their workouts as the people who ran or biked, they burned far more calories over the course of the next several hours. This phenomenon is known as the afterburn – the additional calories your body burns off in the hours and days after a workout. When researchers looked at the metabolic increases after exercise, they found that the increased metabolic effect of aerobics lasted only 30 to 60 minutes. The effects of weight training lasted as long as 48 hours. That's 48 hours during which the body was burning additional fat. Over the long term, both groups lost weight, but those who practised strength training lost only fat, while the runners and bikers lost muscle mass as well. The message: aerobic exercise essentially burns only at the time of the workout. Strength training burns calories long after you leave the gym, while you sleep, and maybe all the way until your next workout. Plus, the extra muscle you build through strength training means that in the long term, your body keeps burning calories at rest just to keep that new muscle alive.

That raises a question. What aspect of strength training creates the long afterburn? Most likely, it's the process of muscle repair. Weight lifting causes your muscle tissues to break down and rebuild themselves at a higher rate than normal. (Muscles are always breaking down and rebuilding; strength training simply accelerates the process.) That breakdown and rebuilding takes a lot of energy and could be what accounts for the long period of calorie burning. In fact, a 2001 Finnish study found that protein synthesis (the process that builds bigger muscles) increases 21 per cent 3 hours after a workout.

The good news is that you don't have to lift like a rugby forward to see the results. A recent Ohio University study found that a short but hard workout had the same effect as longer workouts. Using a circuit of three exercises in a row for 31 minutes, the subjects were still burning more calories than normal 38 hours after the workout. (The Abs Diet Workout is designed along similar principles, to mimic these results.)

As I said earlier, building muscle increases your metabolism so much that you burn up to 50 calories per day per ½ kg/1 lb of muscle you have. The more muscle you have, the easier it is for you to lose fat. That's why one of the components of the plan includes an exercise programme that will help you add the muscle you need to burn fat and reshape your body. And it also points to one of the reasons why you should de-emphasize cardiovascular, aerobic exercise if you want to lose fat: because it depletes your body's store of fat-burning muscle.

Now, before you start thinking I'm some sort of anti-aerobics fanatic, let me clarify a few things: I run almost daily, and I've even completed the New York City Marathon. Aerobic exercise burns calories, it helps control stress, and it improves your cardiovascular fitness. It also helps lower blood pressure and improve your cholesterol profile. If your choice is aerobic exercise or no exercise, for Pete's sake get out there and run. But when it comes to long-term weight management, I'll take gym iron over road rubber any day.

Changing the Way You Eat

FEW THINGS IN our society have failed more often than diets (with the exception of our national football teams). I think there's an explanation for the high failure rate. For one, many diets have revolved around low-fat menus. I'll discuss fat in a later chapter, but one of the problems with low-fat diets is that they can suppress the manufacture of testosterone, the hormone that contributes to the growth of muscle and the burning of fat. When testosterone levels are low, your body stores fat like squirrels store nuts. In one study, men with higher testosterone were 75 per cent less likely to be obese than men with lower levels of testosterone. Many diets also fail because they don't take advantage of the single most powerful nutrient for building muscle and increasing your metabolism: protein.

Protein – in proportion with foods from other groups – works in two primary ways. First, eating more protein cranks up the thermic effect of digestion by as much as one-third. Secondly, protein is also the nutrient that builds calorie-consuming muscle. In effect, you get a double burn – while you're digesting food and later, as it helps build muscle. In the Abs Diet, you'll emphasize protein for these very reasons, but you'll also emphasize the most powerful sources of protein. A Danish study published in the *American Journal of Clinical Nutrition* took a group of men and gave them diets that were high in protein either from pork or from soya. They found that men on the diet higher in animal protein burned 2 per cent more calories during a 24-hour period than men on the soya protein diet, despite the fact that they ate slightly less food. That's 50 calories a day if you're eating a 2,500-calorie diet. In other words, if you want to burn calories, tenderloin is better than tofu.

Changing the Way You Think About the Word *Diet*

HERE'S A TYPICAL diet scenario: you nibble on a piece of toast for breakfast and a sack of baby carrots for lunch, and you figure that puts you well ahead of the calorie-counting game. By dinner, though, you've got so many onion rings jammed into your mouth that you look like Dizzy Gillespie. If you're so restricted in what you can eat, you'll eventually act like a rebellious teen and break the rules. While most diets say 'no' more than your boss at review time, the Abs Diet gives you options. Most diets are about restricting. This one is about fuelling.

For years – or maybe for all your life – you've probably had one notion about what dieting needs to be. Restrict your foods, eat like a supermodel, sweat on the treadmill, and you'll lose fat. In reality, those could be the very reasons why you couldn't lose weight. It's why you gained back what you lost. It's the reason why your speedboat metabolism may have geared down to that of an anchored barge. It's why you don't see much progress when you try new weight-loss programmes. And it's why the only real recipe many diet plans offer is a recipe for pecan-crusted failure. What the Abs Diet will do is reprogramme your circuitry. You'll stop thinking about every calorie and start thinking about how best to burn calories. Once you master that, your body will be equipped with all the tools it needs to strip away fat – and show off your abs.

WHAT THE HECK IS ... DIABETES?

If someone you love has ever struggled with the scourge of diabetes, you know what a devastating disease it can be. Not only is it a leading cause of death in itself, but chances are that this demonic disorder probably contributes to many more deaths by causing heart disease, kidney disease and stroke. Its other complications include blindness, amputation, impotence and nerve damage. It's also highly preventable – and the Abs Diet and the Abs Diet Workout are near-perfect prescriptions.

Diabetes works like this: your digestive system turns brunch into glucose – the form of sugar your body uses for energy – and sends it into the blood-stream. When the glucose hits, your pancreas – a large gland located near your stomach – produces insulin, a hormone, and sends that into the blood-stream as well. Insulin is your body's air traffic controller: it takes command of all your glucose and directs it into your cells, where it can be used for rebuilding muscle, for keeping your heart pumping and your brain thinking, or for doing the macarena (if you're the type to do the macarena, that is).

But over time, bad health habits can take a toll on your flight command centre. Overeating, particularly eating high-glycaemic index foods, floods your body with massive amounts of glucose time and time again. Like any air traffic controller, insulin can become overwhelmed when it's asked to do too much all at one time and, eventually, it burns out. Insulin loses its ability to tell cells how to properly utilize the glucose in your blood – a condition known as insulin resistance. After several years, the pancreas gets fed up with producing all that ineffective insulin and begins to produce less than you need. This is called type 2, or adult-onset, diabetes. (Given that poor diet is the major risk factor, it's no surprise that 80 per cent of people with type 2 diabetes are overweight.) Glucose builds up in the blood, overflows into the urine, and passes out of the body. Thus, the body loses its main source of fuel even though the blood contains large amounts of glucose.

Two bad things happen: first, you start to lose energy, and your body starts to have trouble maintaining itself. You feel fatigue and unusual thirst, and you begin losing weight for no apparent reason; you get sick more often, and injuries are slow to heal, because your body is losing its ability to maintain itself. Secondly, the sugar that is hanging around in your blood begins to damage the tiny blood vessels and nerves throughout your body, particularly in your extremeties and vital organs. Blindness, impotence, numbness and heart damage ensue.

But diabetes is a relatively preventable disease. Exercising and eating right are the two best ways to manage it – and what a coincidence, that's just what this book is intended to teach you to do. So adopt the principles of the Abs Diet and the Abs Diet Workout, and while you're at it, consider these additional steps.

Get mushy. Oats are high in soluble fibre, which may decrease your risk of heart disease, some cancers, diverticulitis and diabetes. Mix it up: eat oat porridge with berries and nuts one day, and have eggs and meat another.

Climb. Yale researchers found that men with insulin resistance – a risk factor for diabetes and heart disease – who exercised on a stairclimber for 45 minutes 4 days a week improved their sensitivity to insulin by 43 per cent in 6 weeks.

Steal from the teacher. Researchers at the National Public Health Institute in Helsinki, Finland, studied the diets of 60,000 men and women over the course of a year and found that individuals who ate apples the most frequently were 12 per cent less likely to die during the course of the study than those who rarely bit into a Cox or Granny Smith. In particular, they cut their risk of diabetes by 27 per cent.

Eat the right carbs. Get to know the glycaemic index, a measure of how quickly the carbohydrates in a particular food are converted to glucose and released into the bloodstream. In a Harvard study, men who ate foods with the lowest indexes, like wholemeal bread, were 37 per cent less likely to develop diabetes than those who ate high-glycaemic index foods, such as white rice.(To find out the glycaemic index of your favourite foods, go to www.glycemicindex.com.)

Eat more E. In the alphabet soup of vitamins, E is the one that may prevent the big D. When Finnish researchers evaluated the diets of 944 men, they found that those with the highest vitamin E intake had a 22 per cent lower risk of diabetes than men with the lowest intake. Vitamin E may also prevent the free radical damage that plays a role in the complications caused by diabetes.

Start wining. In a study of 23,000 twins, researchers found that individuals who had one or two drinks a day were up to 40 per cent less likely to develop diabetes than individuals downing less than one drink daily. Previous research has linked alcohol consumption to increased insulin sensitivity. Just don't overdo the amount you drink. In a separate study, researchers found that binge drinking may increase your risk of colorectal cancer threefold.

Cruise the Mediterranean. Eating a Mediterranean-style diet, that is, whole grains, fresh vegetables and oily fish maximizes your metabolism and slashes diabetes risk. A 2008 study of 13,380 people in the *British Medical Journal* showed that those who adhered closely to a Mediterranean diet had a 35 per cent lower risk of diabetes than those who did not consistently follow such an eating style.

Chapter 4

HOW THE ABS DIET WORKS

What Your Last Meal Is Doing
to Your Body Right Now

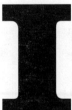N THE CRUDEST FORM, THE WAY IN WHICH
food travels through your body
seems simple. There's one way in
and one way out, and anything left
behind snowballs into a mound of
fat on your gut, over your hips, or under your chin. In
reality, the travel patterns of your breakfast, lunch and
dinner flow more like a motorway intersection than anything else. You've got the traffic jams (clogged arteries)
and the occasional accidents (indigestion), but you also
have a complex network of roads that shuttle nutrients to
and from vital organs and tissues. Your ability to lose
weight and gain muscle largely depends on how and when
you fuel your body to work in that system.

In the previous chapter, I showed how the key to effective weight management was concentrating on your body's calorie burn – not on how effectively you burn calories while exercising but on how effectively you burn calories when you're not exercising. Additionally, I explained a little about how the foods you eat can affect your body's daily calorie burn. Before I explain the how-to's of the Abs Diet, you should know the most important substances and nutrients that affect the way your body processes food.

Protein: The MVP

IN SPORTS, FEW THINGS are as valued as versatility – a cricketer who can bat and bowl, a footballer who attacks as well as he defends. In your body, protein is the most versatile player on your nutrient team. It comes in many forms and does so many things well – all without a £20 million contract.

▶ Protein builds the framework of your body, including muscles, organs, bones and connective tissues.

▶ In the form of enzymes, it helps your body digest food.

▶ As a hormone, it tells your body when to use food as energy and when to store it as fat.

▶ It transports oxygen through your blood to your muscles and organs.

▶ As an antibody, it protects you from illness when viruses and bacteria attack.

So protein is critical for helping your body function at optimum levels. But we've made protein the foundation of the Abs Diet for four other crucial reasons.

1. It tastes good. Juicy steaks. Sliced smoked turkey. Roasted pork loin. Steamed lobster. Peanut butter. The

Abs Diet is built around the foods you crave, so it's a programme you're not going to have to stick to; it's a programme you're going to want to stick to.

2. It burns calories even as you're indulging in it.
Food contains energy in the form of chemical bonds, but your body can't use them in that form. Your body has to break down the food and extract energy from that chemical bond; that process of extracting energy itself requires energy, so your body's burning more calories to do it. That's the thermic effect of eating, as I explained in chapter 3, and protein pushes the thermic effect into high gear. It takes almost two times more energy to break down protein than it does to break down carbohydrates. So when you feed your body a greater amount of protein, your body automatically burns more calories throughout the day. When Arizona State University researchers compared the benefits of a high-protein diet with those of a high-carbohydrate diet, they found that people who ate a high-protein diet burned more than twice as many calories in the hours after their meals as those eating predominantly carbs.

3. It keeps you feeling satisfied. Research has shown that if you base your meals around protein, you'll feel fuller faster. Consider one study in the *European Journal of Clinical Nutrition*. Subjects downed one of four different kinds of shakes – 60 per cent protein, 60 per cent carbohydrate, 60 per cent fat or a mixture of equal amounts of all three. Then they were offered lunch. The subjects who had either the high-protein or mixed-nutrient shakes ate the least for lunch. The shakes they had downed contained the same number of calories, but the protein made them feel fuller and eat less at lunchtime.

4. It builds muscle and keeps your body burning fat all day. Remember, more muscle burns more fat. When you lift and lower weights, you create microscopic tears in your muscles. To repair the tears, protein acts like the Red Cross in a national disaster area. Your body parachutes in new protein to assess the damage and repair the muscle. Proteins fortify the original cell structure by building new muscle fibres.

This whole process through which proteins make new muscle fibres after a workout can last anywhere from 24 to 48 hours. So if you lift weights 3 days a week – triggering proteins to rush in and repair your muscles – your body essentially stays in muscle-building, and thus fat-burning, mode every day.

As you know, protein comes in many forms – such as turkey, beef, fish, nuts and tofu. You want to concentrate on the proteins that best help build your muscles. Research has shows that animal protein builds muscle better than soya or vegetable protein does. So poultry, fish, and lean cuts of beef or pork are a better choice than tofu or other soya-based products. If you're the kind of person who likes to count, you'll want to aim for about 1 gram of protein per ½ kg/1 lb of body weight per day – that's roughly the amount of protein your body can use every day. For a 72.6-kg/11 st 6 lb man, that's 160 grams (g) of protein a day, which would break down into something like this:

3 eggs (18 g)

480 ml/16 fl oz of skimmed milk (16 g)

170 g/6 oz of cottage cheese (28 g)

1 roast beef sandwich (28 g)

75 g/2½ oz of peanuts (16 g)

230 g/8 oz of chicken breast (54 g)

Combine those four reasons – an easy and delicious eating plan, more calorie burn, less calorie intake and more fat-burning muscle – and you can easily see how a high-protein diet translates into weight loss. In a Danish study, researchers put 65 subjects on a 12 per cent protein diet, a 25 per cent protein diet, or no diet (the control group). In the first two groups, the same percentage of calories – about 30 per cent – came from fat. While the low-protein dieters lost an average of more than 5 kg/11 lb, the high-protein subjects lost an average of 9 kg/20 lb and ate fewer calories than the low-protein group.

The more amazing statistic wasn't how much they lost but where they lost it: the high-protein dieters also lost twice as much abdominal fat. One reason may be that a high-protein diet helps your body control its levels of cortisol, a stress hormone that causes fat to converge in the abdominal region.

Fat: Underrated, Understand?

WHEN YOU THINK of fat, you probably think of foods that have a lot of fat – or people who do. After a few years with some extra weight, the only thing you know about fat is that you're tired of it and want to get rid of it for ever. But it's probably one of your body's most misunderstood dietary nutrients, stemming from a widely held but misguided belief that fat should take much of the blame for our obesity epidemic.

In the 1980s, the government released nutritional guidelines that essentially said we should base our diets on potatoes, rice, cereal and pasta and minimize the foods with a lot of fat and protein. That gave way to the idea that fat makes you fat. And that gave way to a new breed of diets that said if you limit the fat in what you eat, you'll limit the fat that exercises squatter's rights on your gut. But that line of thinking didn't hold up when researchers tried to find links between low-fat diets and obesity.

In 1998, for example, two prominent obesity researchers estimated that if you took only 10 per cent of your calories from fat,
you'd lose 16 grams of fat a day – a loss of 22.6 kg/3 st 8 lb in a
year. But when a Harvard epidemiologist, Walter Willett, tried to
find evidence that this occurred, he couldn't find any link between
people who lost weight and the fact that they were on a low-fat
diet. In fact, in some studies lasting a year or more, groups of
people showed weight *gains* on low-fat diets. Willett speculated
that there was a mechanism responsible for this: when the body
is on a low-fat diet for a long period, it stops losing weight.

Part of the reason our bodies rebel against low-fat diets is that
we need fat. For instance, fat plays a vital role in the delivery of
vitamins A, D, E and K, nutrients stored in fatty tissue and the
liver until your body needs them. Fat also helps produce testosterone, which helps trigger muscle growth. And fat, like protein,
helps keep you satisfied and controls your appetite. In fact, if we've
learned anything about weight loss over the past several years, it's
that reducing your fat intake doesn't necessarily do a darn thing
to decrease your body fat. One small study, for instance, compared
a high-carbohydrate diet and a high-fat diet. The researchers
found that the group with the high-fat diet experienced less muscle
loss than the other group. The researchers theorized that muscle
protein was being spared by the higher-fat diet because fatty acids,
more so than carbs, were being harnessed and used for energy.

The truth is that reasonable amounts of fat can actually help
you lose weight. In a study from the *International Journal of Obesity*, researchers at Boston's Brigham and Women's Hospital and
Harvard Medical School put 101 overweight people on either a
low-fat diet (fat was 20 per cent of the total calories) or a moderate
-fat diet (35 per cent of calories) and followed them for 18 months.
Both groups lost weight at first, but after a year and a half, the
moderate-fat group had lost an average of 4 kg/9 lb per person,
whereas the low-fat dieters had *gained* 2.75 kg/6 lb. The results

suggest that a healthy amount of fat is a factor in keeping your weight under control.

Here's a primer on the fats in your life.

Trans fat: BAD. You won't find trans fatty acids listed on most food labels, even though there are more than 40,000 packaged foods that contain this type of fat. You won't find it listed because it's so bad for you that food manufacturers have fought for years to keep it off ingredient labels. In 2003, the US Food and Drug Administration finally adopted regulations requiring manufacturers to include trans fat content on their packaging, and the regulations will be phased in over the next few years. In the UK, food manufacturers are not, as yet, required to list trans fats on labels, but the European Commission is due to review its Nutritional Labelling Directive in the near future. For now, you have to be a smart food consumer to spot where the danger lies.

Trans fats were invented by grocery manufacturers in the 1950s as a way of appealing to our natural cravings for fatty foods. But there's nothing natural about trans fats – they're cholesterol-raising, heart-weakening, diabetes-causing, belly-building chemicals that, for the most part, didn't even exist until the middle of the last century, and some studies have linked them to premature death. In one Harvard study, researchers found that getting just 3 per cent of your daily calories from trans fats increased your risk of heart disease by 50 per cent. Three per cent of your daily calories equals about 7 grams of trans fats – that's roughly the amount in a single order of french fries.

To understand what trans fats are, picture a bottle of vegetable oil and a packet of margarine. At room temperature, the vegetable oil is a liquid, the margarine a solid. Now, if you baked biscuits using vegetable oil, they'd be pretty greasy. And who would want to buy a biscuit swimming in oil? So to create biscuits – and cakes, crisps (potato chips), pies, muffins, doughnuts, waffles and many, many other foods we consume daily – manufacturers heat the oil to very high temperatures and infuse it with hydrogen. That hydrogen bonds with the oil to create an entirely new form of fat – trans fat – that stays solid at room temperature. Vegetable oil becomes margarine. And now foods that might normally be healthy – but maybe not as tasty – become fat bombs.

Since these trans fats don't exist in nature, your body has a hell of a time processing them. Once consumed, trans fats are free to cause all sorts of mischief inside you. They raise the number of LDL (bad) cholesterol particles in your bloodstream and lower your HDL (good) cholesterol. They also raise blood levels of other lipoproteins; the more lipoprotein you have in your bloodstream, the greater your risk of heart disease. Increased consumption of trans fats has also been linked to increased risk of diabetes and cancer.

Yet trans fats are added to a shocking number of foods. They appear on food labels as PARTIALLY HYDROGENATED OIL – usually vegetable or palm oil. Go look in your larder and freezer right now, and you won't believe how many foods include them. Crackers. Popcorn. Biscuits. Cheese spreads. Confectionery bars. Frozen waffles. Stuffing. Even foods you might assume are healthy – like bran muffins, cereals and non-dairy creamers – are often loaded with trans fats. And because they hide in foods that look like they're low in fat, these fats are making you unhealthy without your even knowing it.

HOW TO CHOOSE A MULTIVITAMIN

Multivitamins are good insurance for the day you don't get the daily maximum amount of nutrients. Look for one with a concentration of chromium and vitamins B_6 and B_{12}. Chromium improves your body's ability to convert amino acids into muscle. A University of Maryland study found that men who exercised regularly and took 200 micrograms of chromium a day added more muscle and lost significantly more body fat than those not taking the supplement. Also, since hard workouts deplete your B vitamins, it's good to find vitamins with high doses, like Wellman multivitamins, which has megadoses of vitamins B_6 and B_{12}, plus your entire daily allowance of endurance-boosting zinc.

Take control of your trans fat intake. Check the ingredient labels on all the packaged foods you buy, and if you see PARTIALLY HYDROGENATED OIL on the label, consider finding an alternative. Even foods that seem bad for you can have healthy versions: McCain's french fries, Ruffles Natural reduced-fat crisps, Finn Crisp crackers and Green & Black's chocolate bars are just a few of the 'bad for you' snacks that are actually free of trans fats. And remember – the higher up on the ingredients' list PARTIALLY HYDRO-GENATED OIL is, the worse the food is for you. You might not be able to avoid trans fats entirely, but you can choose foods with a min-imal amount of the stuff.

The other way to avoid trans fats is to avoid ordering fried foods. Because trans fats spoil less easily than natural fats and are easier to ship and store, almost all fried commercial foods are now fried in trans fats rather than natural oils. Fish and chips, tortillas, fried chicken – all of it is packed with belly-building trans fats. Order food baked or grilled whenever possible. And avoid fast-food joints, where nearly every food option is loaded with trans fats; drive-through restaurants ought to come com-plete with drive-through cardiology clinics.

For more on trans fats – where they come from, how they act inside your body, and how to fight back, see the Special Report on page 143. In the meantime:

AVOID

Margarine

Fried foods

Commercially manufactured baked goods

Any food with PARTIALLY HYDROGENATED OIL on its list of ingredients

Saturated fat: BAD. Saturated fats are naturally occurring fats found in meat and dairy products. The problem with satur-ated fats is that when they enter your body, they tend to do the same thing they did when they were in a pig's or cow's body: rather than be burned for energy, they're more likely to be stored as fat in your flanks, in your ribs, even – ugh – in your loin. In fact, they seem to have more of a 'storage effect' than other fats. A new study from Johns Hopkins University suggests that the amount of saturated fat in your diet may be directly proportional to the amount of fat surrounding your abdominal muscles. Researchers analysed the diets of 84 people and performed an MRI scan on each of them to measure fat. Those whose diets included the highest rates of saturated fat also had the most abdominal fat. Saturated fats also raise cholesterol levels, so they increase your risk of heart disease and some types of cancer.

I don't want you to eliminate saturated fats entirely; they're found in most animal products, and those food products are

---

ABS DIET SUCCESS STORY

'THE ABS DIET HELPED ME CHEAT DEATH!'

Name: Dan Shea

Age: 40

Height: 1.7 m/5'7"

Starting weight: 103 kg/16 st 2 lb

Six weeks later: 94 kg/14 st 11 lb

Dan Shea had seen what happens to a man who doesn't take charge of his weight and his health, and he didn't want it to happen to him. His own dad – a once-fit airborne ranger who used to be in incredible shape – was now, aged 70, on the verge of losing a foot to diabetes. Shea wanted to plot a different course: 'I want to be skiing when I'm 70,' he says.

But at 40 years old, 1.7 m/5 ft 7 in, and 103 kg/16 st 2 lb, Shea knew he had to make a change – a 27 kg/4-st change. He had a 13-year-old daughter he wanted to watch grow up, and at the rate he was going, he was a heart attack waiting to happen. So he started the Abs Diet and immediately took to it. He realized he wasn't eating enough breakfast and also realized the importance

important for the Abs Diet for other reasons (the calcium in dairy products, the protein in meat). But I do want you to consume the low-fat and leaner versions of meat and dairy products. You want the nutritional benefit from one part of the food without high amounts of saturated fat.

AVOID

Fatty cuts of red meat

Whole-milk dairy products

Polyunsaturated fats: GOOD. There are two types of poly-unsaturated fats: omega-3s and omega-6s. You've probably heard of omega-3 fatty acids. They're the fats found in fish, and a diet high in omega-3s has been shown to help protect the

of eating often – making sure he had a mid-morning snack consisting of a couple of the Powerfoods. 'Even though I wasn't hungry, I ate it,' he says. 'It was like fighting years of dietary knowledge to have that mid-morning snack. I wasn't hungry yet, but if I hadn't eaten, I'd have been starving at lunch.'

But his biggest affection is for the Abs Diet smoothies that he makes with low-fat yogurt, low-fat milk, some fruit and a scoop of protein powder. 'Best damn thing on the planet, as good as eating Häagen-Dazs,' Shea says. 'For fun, I'd layer it with a couple of tablespoons of fat-free, sugar-free whipped topping. My life is all about smoothies now. It's my snack of choice – really my meal of choice. If I could have a blender in my office, I'd have them three times a day.'

Shea lost 9 kg/nearly 20 lb on the plan and has made the Abs Diet his regular eating and nutritional plan as he strives for his goal of 75 kg/11 st 11 lb. 'I look great, or so my wife tells me. My trousers are much looser, and I need a new belt. I tuck in my shirts now. I walk taller somehow, stand taller. My confidence level has been boosted. In fact, I had an interview for a position for which I was way underqualified, yet I was short-listed and came quite close to getting it, based largely on my strength of presence,' Shea says. 'I've lost in my gut and butt, but mainly my man breasts are now less Dolly Parton and more Gwyneth Paltrow. I know this is a great plan, and I know I'm going to reach my goal. I'm in it for the long haul, and this is a plan that is easy to do for the long term.'

heart from cardiovascular disease. That's plenty enough reason to include seafood in your diet. But new evidence suggests that this type of fat can actually help you control your weight. In one study, subjects who took in 6 grams a day of fish oil supplements burned more fat during the course of a day than those who went without. Researchers suspect that a diet high in omega-3s actually alters the body's metabolism and spurs it to burn fat more efficiently.

Even more recently, a study in Iceland found that dieters who ate salmon felt fuller two hours later than those who either didn't eat oily fish or ate cod, a fish with a very small amount of omega-3s. The researchers found that eating foods high in omega-3s increased blood levels of leptin, a hormone that promotes satiety.

Now, you can take fish oil supplements if you want, but you'll miss the muscle-building protein benefits of real fish. The fish with the highest levels of omega-3s are the fish you probably enjoy the most already – salmon and tuna, to name two. (To see where your favourite fish falls in the omega-3 sweepstakes, see the chart on the opposite page.) In addition to being packed with heart-healthy, fat-burning omega-3s, fish is also a great source of lean, muscle-building protein.

There's another amazing, secret Powerfood that bodybuilders know about but you may have never even heard of: flaxseed. Flax is a seldom-used grain that's *loaded* with omega-3s as well as cholesterol-busting fibre. You'll find flaxseeds and flaxseed oil in most health food stores. Grab it! I keep ground flaxseed in the fridge, and I toss it on breakfast cereals, into smoothies, and on top of ice cream. It's got a mild nutty flavour you'll like. It crushes cholesterol with its omega-3s, it adds artery-scouring fibre to your diet, and it might just be your best weapon against fat.

Omega-6 fatty acids also help lower bad cholesterol and raise good cholesterol. They're found in vegetable oils, meat, eggs and dairy products. They're so common to so many foods, in fact, that only those of you currently shipwrecked on deserted islands living off flotsam and jetsam need worry about not getting enough in your diet.

EAT MORE

Fish

Flaxseed and flaxseed oil

Monounsaturated fats: GOOD. Monounsaturated fats are found in nuts, olives, peanuts, avocados and olive and rapeseed (canola) oils. Like omega-3s, these fats help reduce cholesterol levels and protect against heart disease, but they also help you burn fat; in one study, researchers found that the body burns more fat in the 5 hours following a meal high in monos than after a meal rich in saturated fats.

Monounsaturated fats will not only lower your cholesterol and

SEAFOOD WITH THE HIGHEST OMEGA-3 CONTENT

All data are for 90-g/3-oz servings (except for sardines, which is for 105 g/ 3¾ oz). Aim for a total of 1 gram (g) of omega-3s per day.

TYPE OF FISH	OMEGA-3 CONTENT	PREPARED
Sardines	2.3 g	Brine-packed can
Salmon	2.0 g	Poached
Mackerel	1.8 g	Grilled
Tuna	1.4 g	Grilled
Trout	1.1 g	Grilled
Shark	1.1 g	Grilled
Swordfish	1.1 g	Grilled
Oysters	0.5 g	Boiled
Tuna	0.07 g	250-g/9-oz water-packed can

help you burn off your tummy but will also help you eat less. Penn State researchers found that men who ate mashed potatoes prepared with oil high in monounsaturated fats like olive oil felt fuller longer than when they ate mash made with polyunsaturated fats like vegetable oil.

Carbohydrates: A Bad Rap

WITH THE BEATINGS that carbohydrates have taken over the past few years, it's a wonder that bread isn't protected by the Endangered Species Act. Everywhere I look, I see people eating burgers without buns, ordering spaghetti and meatballs – hold the spaghetti – or bragging about their all-bacon-all-the-time diet. While it's clear that protein and fat have tremendous nutritional benefits, it's unfair – and unhealthy – to kick carbohydrates off the dietary island.

With more and more evidence showing that a high-carbohydrate diet helps promote fat storage (unless you run marathons), it's becoming more accepted that low-carbohydrate diets work in helping people control weight. A 2002 study in the journal *Metabolism* confirmed that very stance. Researchers at the University of Connecticut found that subjects who ate only 46 grams of carbohydrates a day – about 8 per cent of calories – lost 3.2 kg/7 lb of fat and gained 900 g/2 lb of muscle in 6 weeks. And they did it while downing a satisfying 2,337 calories a day. But you can make a major mistake by eliminating carbohydrates entirely. Many carbohydrates – like fruits, vegetables, whole grains and beans – help protect you against cancer and other diseases, and some carbs also contain fibre, which helps you lose and control weight.

Traditionally, the confusion about carbohydrates has centred around finding ways to classify them and figuring out which ones are better for your body. It used to be that we thought of carbohydrates only by their molecular structure – either simple or complex. Simple indicates a carb with one or two sugar molecules – things like sucrose (table sugar), fructose (in fruit) and lactose (in dairy products). Complex carbohydrates are ones that include more than two sugar molecules – like pasta, rice, bread and potatoes. The flaw is that you can't generalize and say a carbohydrate is good or bad for you based simply on its molecular structure. For example, an apple contains nutrients and helps keep you lean; sugar does not. Both are simple carbs, but they're hardly comparable in nutritional value.

Instead, the way to decide what carbohydrates are best for you stems from how your body reacts to the carbohydrates chemically. One of the tools that nutritionists use today is the glycaemic index (GI). The GI assigns numbers to foods that indicate how quickly a food turns into glucose. High-GI foods – ones that are quickly digested and turned to glucose – are generally less nutritionally sound than low-GI choices.

Another term for glucose is blood sugar. The presence of sugar in your blood causes your body to produce the hormone insulin. Insulin's job is to move the sugar you're not using for energy out of your bloodstream and store it in your body. Here's where the GI comes into effect: foods with a high GI (like pasta, bread, white rice and Snickers bars) are digested quickly, flooding your bloodstream with sugar. Insulin rushes in and says, 'Whoa, what do I do with all of this?' Whatever glucose isn't immediately burned for energy quickly starts getting stored as fat. What's worse is that if you eat a carb with a high GI in combination with fat – bread with butter, for example – none of the fat you eat can be burned for energy either, because your bloodstream is so flooded with sugar. Insulin does such a good job of turning this new blood sugar into fat, in fact, that soon your blood sugar begins to drop, and you know what that means: you're hungry again.

If you eat a meal with a low GI (like a balanced dinner of chicken, high-fibre vegetables and brown rice), the food is digested more slowly. Your blood sugar rises only incrementally, and that slow digestion means that glucose is available as energy for hours and hours. That means you have hours and hours to burn off the blood sugar. Insulin doesn't need to rush in and turn the sugar into fat; it can use the sugar slowly for other construction projects, like building and repairing muscle. Moreover, because your blood sugar levels stay even, you don't turn ravenously hungry just a few hours after eating. You build more muscle, you store less fat, you have more energy, and you keep your appetite under control.

INSULIN: THE TWO-FACED HORMONE

The hormone insulin is like your pack-rat grandmother: it likes to store stuff. The only problem is that it's also as schizophrenic as Dr Jekyll. Sometimes it makes your muscles grow; sometimes it makes your fat cells grow.

Different foods create different insulin responses. Foods that have high-glycaemic index rankings (including white bread, most cereals, grapes and bananas) dump a lot of sugar into your bloodstream soon after eating, causing insulin levels to spike. In this case, insulin works quickly to turn that blood sugar into fat.

Some foods, though, cause a different reaction. Dairy products – milk, yogurt, ice cream – create dramatic insulin surges without the corresponding effect on blood sugar. You also get this insulin response from some foods that are virtually carbohydrate-free, such as beef and fish, which have hardly any effect on blood sugar. When blood sugar remains relatively constant, it allows insulin to use the nutrients in your blood to build and repair cells, including muscle tissue.

That's why the Abs Diet centres around high-fibre, nutrient-dense foods that are also the ones thought to be most useful for weight control. Most are moderate to high protein, some are high in dairy calcium, and those that are carb-based emphasize fibre and other important nutrients.

(By the way, if all this talk about blood sugar and insulin reminds you of a certain health problem – diabetes – then you were obviously paying attention in health class. Continuing to flood your bloodstream with high levels of sugar, followed by high levels of insulin, eventually trains your body to become less efficient at processing these blood sugars. That's called insulin resistance, which is another term for diabetes. It is a terrible, terrible disease – and it is also highly preventable. In a Harvard study, men who ate foods with the lowest GIs, like wholemeal bread, were 37 per cent less likely to develop diabetes than those who ate high-GI foods, such as white rice. For more information on battling diabetes, see our Health Bulletin on page 66.

It's hard to generalize about which carbs are high on the GI list and which are low, because the glycaemic index is simply a measure of time – that is, how long it takes 50 grams of the food's carbohydrates to turn into blood sugar, regardless of serving size. It's a measure, for instance, of the carb-to-sugar conversion time for a whole apple or watermelon, but it doesn't tell you how much carb is in *one serving* of the food. Nobody eats a *whole* watermelon, anyway.

That's why the latest advancement in food science is to look at a meal's *glycaemic load* (GL). The GL considers both the GI of a food and the amount of carbs in one serving of that food. It helps you gauge the glycaemic effect, or the projected elevation of blood glucose, that food will cause.

The higher a food's GL, the more it will cause your blood sugar to spike, and the less control you'll have over your energy levels and your appetite. But considering the GL is only one aspect of creating a balanced diet. 'It's better to have a high-GL diet than one full of saturated fat,' says Jennie Brand-Miller, PhD, professor of human nutrition at the University of Sydney and author of the *International Table of Glycemic Index and Glycemic Load*. 'Aiming for the lowest GL possible is not a good move because that means you'll be eating too little carbohydrate and too much fat – probably saturated fat.' Instead, to maintain your body's best glycaemic response, base your meals around foods with GLs of 19 or less and aim for a GL of less than 120 for the whole day.

Sounds confusing? It doesn't need to be. The Abs Diet Power-foods and the Abs Diet recipes all have low to moderate glycaemic loads. All you have to do is follow the plan. And on those occasions when you are stuck and need to choose between two or more foods, refer to the chart on page 292.

Calcium: The Future of Fat Fighting

YOU'VE SEEN MORE than enough milk moustaches to know that calcium strengthens your bones, but did you know that calcium can also firm up your gut? Researchers at Harvard Medical School showed that those who ate three servings of dairy a day – which in conjunction with other foods provides about 1,200 milligrams of calcium (about the daily recommendation) – were 60 per cent less likely to be overweight. In studies at the University of Tennessee, researchers put subjects on diets that were 500 calories a day less than what they were used to eating. Yup, the subjects lost weight – about ½ kg/1 lb of fat a week. But when researchers put another set of subjects on the same diet but added dairy to their meals, their fat loss doubled, to around 1 kg/2 lb a week. Same calorie intake, double the fat loss.

Calcium seems to limit the amount of new fat your body can make, according to the University of Tennessee research team. In another study conducted at the same lab, men who added three servings of yogurt a day to their diets lost 61 per cent more body fat and 81 per cent more stomach fat over 12 weeks than men who didn't eat yogurt. A study in Hawaii found that teenagers with the highest calcium intakes were thinner and leaner than those getting less calcium.

Some researchers speculate that dairy calcium helps fight fat because it increases the thermic effect of eating – in other words, you burn more calories digesting calcium-rich foods than you would if you ate something with equal calories but no calcium. That's one reason why calcium supplements, though good for bone-building and other bodily functions, don't have the same effect as dairy – fewer calories to digest, so fewer calories to burn.

And calcium has its benefits beyond stronger bones and leaner bodies. After analysing data from 47,000 men involved in the Health Professional's Follow-Up Study, Harvard researchers found that men whose diets included 700 to 800 milligrams of the mineral a day were up to 50 per cent less likely to develop some forms of colon cancer than men whose diets contained less than 500 milligrams. For best effect, aim for about 1,200 milligrams (mg) of calcium per day.

The Abs Diet-recommended calcium-rich foods are:

▶ 30 g/1 oz grated Parmesan cheese (314 mg)

▶ 170 ml/6 oz large-curd cottage cheese (126 mg)

▶ 240 ml/8 fl oz low-fat yogurt (415 mg)

▶ 240 ml/8 fl oz skimmed milk (264 mg)

▶ 30 g/1 oz (2.5-cm/1-in cube) Gruyère cheese (224 mg)

▶ 30 g/1 oz (1 slice) Cheddar cheese (204 mg)

▶ 30 g/1 oz mozzarella cheese (143 mg)

▶ 1 scoop (28 g) whey powder protein (110 mg)

WHAT THE HECK ARE . . . CANCER CELLS?

Cancer is a scourge that can strike any of us at any time in life. It can hit in the places we think about and care about on a daily basis – the skin, the lungs, the brain – or in obscure places we don't even understand, like the pancreas, the kidneys or the lymphatic system.

Simply put, cancer develops when cells in one part of the body begin to grow out of control. As children, our cells are constantly dividing, creating the new cells that help us grow. Once we reach adulthood, that cell growth stops, for the most part. Once we reach our genetically programmed height and weight, cells in most parts of the body divide only to replace worn-out or dying cells or to repair injuries. (That's why there's no mid-thirties growth spurt, much as we may wish for it.)

But cancer cells act like kids – they keep growing, dividing and multiplying, outliving our normal cells and interfering with the various functions of the body. The most common type of cancer among men is prostate cancer (the prostate is the gland located behind the scrotum that produces most of our seminal fluid). The most common type of cancer among women is breast cancer. The former results in 24,000 new cases each year, the latter 40,000.

We don't fully understand what causes cancer, but we do know some of the risk factors: obesity, low-fibre diets, smoking, heavy alcohol use, overexposure to the sun and exposure to radiation and other toxins are among the biggest dangers. Additionally, there's a strong link between heredity and cancer; if one or more close relatives has suffered a bout of the disease, you're at increased risk of cancer in general and for that specific form of cancer in particular.

I'd like to tell you that the Abs Diet is a magic bullet against cancer, but I can't; while dietary changes and exercise can dramatically decrease your risk of heart disease, stroke and especially diabetes, cancer remains a bit more elusive. Still, by adopting the principles of the Abs Diet, you'll automatically decrease your risk of many forms of cancer, because you'll decrease your weight and increase your fibre intake. In the meantime, you can also follow these additional tips to slash your risk even more.

Toss in the tomatoes. Tomatoes are one of the best sources of lycopene, a nutrient that has been shown to inhibit the growth of prostate cancer cells. In fact, researchers say that two to four servings of tomatoes a week can cut your prostate cancer risk by 34 per cent. (Even better news: lycopene isn't diminished by cooking, so pasta sauce and pizza will strike a blow against the disease as well.)

Colour your plate. A 14-year study found that men whose diets were highest in fruits and vegetables had a 70 per cent lower risk of digestive-tract cancers.

Order the Chilean red. Chilean cabernet sauvignon is 38 per cent higher than French wine in flavonols – compounds called antioxidants that help deter cancer.

Try the cheese platter. A large-scale study of 120,000 women found that premenopausal women who consumed a lot of dairy products, especially low-fat and fat-free ones, ran a lower risk of breast cancer. Pay attention, men: you can get breast cancer, too. And Harvard researchers have found that men with diets high in calcium were up to 50 per cent less likely to develop some forms of colon cancer.

Squeeze a carrot. One 240-ml/8-fl oz glass of pure pressed carrot juice gives you 700 per cent of your daily recommended allowance for beta-carotene (and only 70 calories). Beta-carotene has been linked in several studies to a lower risk of cancer.

Bite the broccoli. It contains a compound called indole-3-carbinol, which has been shown to fight various forms of cancer. Don't like broccoli? Try daikon, an Asian radish that looks like a big white carrot. It's a distant cousin.

Serve the salmon. Or any other fish high in omega-3 fatty acids. Omega-3s can help mollify your cancer risk.

Order drinks with a twist. According to University of Arizona research, lemon zest and orange zest contain d-limonene, an antioxidant that can reduce your risk of skin cancer by up to 30 per cent if you consume quantities as small as 1 tablespoon per week.

Go green. In a recent Rutgers University study, mice given green tea had 51 per cent fewer incidences of skin cancer than control mice. Green tea is another great source of cancer-fighting antioxidants.

Get a D. Foods high in vitamin D, like low-fat milk, help detoxify cancer-causing chemicals released during the digestion of high-fat foods, according to a study at the University of Texas Southwestern Medical Center.

Be Popeye. Japanese researchers found that neoxanthin, a compound in spinach, was successful at preventing the growth of prostate cancer cells.

Show yourself the whey. Whey protein is a great source of cysteine, a major building block of the prostate cancer-fighting agent glutathione.

Eat the whole grain. Wholegrain carbohydrates are a great source of fibre. European researchers found that men with the highest daily intakes of fibre also had a 40 per cent lower risk of developing colon cancer.

Chapter 5

A SIX-PACK IN 6 WEEKS

A Week-by-Week Guide
to How Your Body Will Change

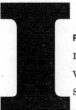**F YOU FLIP THROUGH THIS BOOK, YOU'LL** meet some of the men and women who went on the Abs Diet – and succeeded.

Patrick Austin lost 13.6 kg/ 30 lb, half of it in just the first 2 weeks. Now he can't wait to take off his shirt at the beach.

John Betson turned a flabby 91-cm/36-in waist into a solid 81 cm/32 in and saw his abs for the first time in years.

And Jessica Guff stopped skipping meals – and started wearing skimpier tops.

For Bill Stanton, the turnaround was an eye-opener: 'I'd been lifting weights all my life, but just by changing my diet, my body got leaner and stronger than ever. Guys at the gym even accuse me of being on steroids!'

Everyone's body is different, and everybody who tries this plan will have a different starting point. But based on the scientific research I've outlined, you can expect an average loss of up to 9 kg/20 lb of fat on the 6-week plan and, for men, a gain of 1.8 to 2.75 kg/4 to 6 lb of muscle (about half that amount for women). For the average man, that's enough of a transformation to have your abs show. One of the bigger challenges, however, is monitoring your progress on the plan. Here's a look at the four major measurements you can use to see just how effectively the Abs Diet will work for you.

Weight. It's the most straightforward. The heavier you are, the more at risk you are for disease and the less fit you are. It's a good measuring stick to gauge how well you're progressing on your diet, but it's incomplete in that it doesn't take into account the amount of muscle you're going to develop over the course of

---

ABS DIET SUCCESS STORY

'I CUT MY BODY FAT IN HALF!'

Name: James Schellman

Age: 26

Height: 1.72 m/5'8"

Starting weight: 74.4 kg/11 st 10 lb

Six weeks later: 70.8 kg/11 st 2 lb

A former professional athlete and an active guy who snowboards 60 days a year, James Schellman didn't feel like he needed to lose that much weight. But then a series of nagging injuries started hampering his active lifestyle, and he packed on an extra 4.5 kg/10 lb of tummy flab. Schellman could have blamed the weight gain and injuries on getting older, but that wasn't his style. 'I didn't want to slow down,' he says, 'but I knew I needed a change.' So he went on the Abs Diet to improve his condition and increase

the plan. Muscle weighs about 20 per cent more than fat so even a dramatic fat loss may not translate into a dramatic drop in body weight.

Body mass index (BMI). The BMI is a formula that takes into consideration your height and your weight, and gives you an indication of whether you're overweight, obese, or in good shape. To calculate your BMI, divide your weight in kilograms by your height in metres squared. For example, let's say you're 1.83 m (6 ft) tall and weigh 90 kg (14 st 4 lb). First you square your height.

$1.83 \times 1.83 = 3.348$

Now we divide your weight by this number.

$90 \div 3.348 = 26.9$

That's not terrible. A BMI between 25 and 30 indicates you're overweight. Over 30 signifies obesity.

This measurement, too, has flaws. It doesn't take into account muscle mass, and it also leaves out another important factor –

his muscle tone. Besides, Schellman says, 'I figured I need to look good for my wife.'

During the plan, Schellman lost 3.6 kg/8 lb. But the most significant transformation: he cut his body fat from 18 to 11 per cent.

Schellman has always enjoyed eating healthily, but adjusting to the Abs Diet paid off. 'Before the plan, I ate about four meals a day and counted calories. And with this one, I ate six times a day and let calories go by the wayside,' he says. By basing meals around the delicious Powerfoods, 'I didn't have to worry about the calories I was taking in.'

Schellman, who is used to spending a lot of time in the gym, credits the Abs Diet Workout and its emphasis on lower-body exercises for making him stronger and leaner and helping him burn off that burgeoning belly. 'I have seen stomach fat decrease. I can clearly see some of the muscles [in my abdomen],' he says. 'The plan has been a huge success – I've seen an increase in my overall body strength, an increase in my motivation, an increase in my self-esteem, and an increase in my well-being.'

weight distribution, that is, where most of the fat on your body resides. But BMI can give you a pretty good idea of how serious your weight problem is.

Waist-to-hip ratio. Researchers have begun using waist size and its relationship to hip size as a more definitive way to determine your health risk. This is considered more important than BMI because of that visceral fat I talked about earlier – the fat that pushes your waist out in front of you. Because abdominal fat is the most dangerous fat, a lower waist-to-hip ratio means fewer health risks. To figure out your waist-to-hip ratio, measure your waist at your tummy button and your hips at the widest point (around your bottom). Divide your waist by your hips. For example, if your hips measure 101.6 cm/40 in and your waist at tummy button level measures 96.5 cm/38 in, your waist-to-hip ratio is 0.95.

$$96.5 \div 101.6 = 0.95 \text{ or } 38 \div 40 = 0.95$$

That's not bad, but it's not ideal. You want a waist-to-hip ratio of 0.92 or lower. If you were to lose just 5 cm/2 in off your waist – something you can do in just 2 weeks with the Abs Diet – you'd find yourself in the fit range.

$$91.5 \div 101.6 = 0.90 \text{ or } 36 \div 40 = 0.90$$

Body fat percentage. Though this is the most difficult for the average man to measure because it requires a bit of technology, it's the most useful in terms of gauging how well your diet plan is working. That's because it takes into consideration not just weight but how much of your weight is fat. Many gyms offer body fat measurements through such methods as body fat scales or calipers that measure the folds of fat at several points on your body. See your local gym for what options they offer. Or try an at-home body fat calculator. If you want a simple low-tech test (and this isn't as accurate as what the electronic versions will give you), try this simple exercise: sit in a chair with your knees bent and your feet flat on the floor. Using your thumb and index finger, gently pinch the skin on top of your right thigh. Measure the thickness of the pinched skin with a ruler. If it's 1.9 cm/¾ in or less, you have about 14 per cent body fat – ideal for a guy, quite fit for a woman. If it's 2.5 cm/1 in, you're probably closer to 18 per cent fat, which is a tad high for a man but desirable for a woman. If you pinch more than 2.5 cm/1 in, you could be at increased risk of diabetes and heart disease.

This last measurement can be the most significant because it'll really help give you a sense of how well you're sticking to a plan. As you see your body fat percentage decrease, you'll see an increase in the amount of visible muscle. Experts say that in order for your abs to show, your body fat needs to be between 8 and 12 per cent. For the average slightly overweight man, that means cutting body fat by about half.

Before you start the plan, it's important to record some of these measurements so that you'll know how far you're progressing. Take one baseline measurement, and then remeasure as needed for motivation. I'd recommend measuring every 2 weeks. That'll be enough time to see significant differences to propel you through the next 2 weeks. (Measure body fat percentage only at the beginning and end of the plan, unless you have easy access to a measurement system.) Any sooner than that, and you're focusing too much on numbers rather than process.

MEASUREMENT	START	END OF WEEK 2	END OF WEEK 4	FINISH
Weight				
BMI				
Waist-to-hip ratio				
Body fat percentage*				

*Make sure to have the same person administer body fat readings using the same method to ensure consistency.

As with any diet plan, it's also important to develop some kind of quantitative goal – your ideal weight, waist size or percentage of body fat. This chart will help you figure out where you are and where you need to go.

I don't mean to hit you with more numbers than a fantasy football nerd. In fact, it might be easiest to simply focus on one number – six – so that the others will fall into place. When you start to see those six abdominal muscles, it'll mean that everything else has decreased – your weight, your BMI, your waist-to-hip ratio and your body fat percentage. This 6-week plan will get you there. Here's what you can expect from going on the diet.

WEEKS	WHAT TO EXPECT	WHAT THEY SAY
1–2	A significant weight loss as your body adjusts to a new approach to eating. Some may see losses up to 5.4 kg/12 lb in the first 2 weeks (especially if you're walking, or otherwise active, each day), but 2.25–3.6 kg/5 to 8 lb will be average.	**PATRICK AUSTIN LOST 6.8 KG/15 LB IN JUST THE FIRST COUPLE OF WEEKS ON THE ABS DIET.** *'I haven't gone shirtless on the beach in years,'* he says. *'This year, I'm going to be shirtless.'* Read more about Patrick's success on page 116.
3–4	By integrating a modest amount of strength training into your routine, you'll start to feel your body change because your metabolism is working hard. You'll notice an additional drop in weight (most likely averaging another 2.25 to 3.6 kg/5 to 8 lb), but you'll also notice significant changes in your shape.	**BRIAN ARCHIQUETTE LOST 11.3 KG/25 LB IN 6 WEEKS.** *'I definitely have more energy and a more positive outlook on life,'* he says. Read more about Brian's success on page 176.
5–6	After 2 weeks of exercise, your body is primed to make a significant push to drop more fat while also gaining muscle mass. You'll notice that your upper body is more toned and that your waist and other fatty parts of your body are smaller. Depending on your starting point, this is where you'll begin to see abs.	**JOHN BETSON DECREASED HIS BODY FAT FROM 23 PER CENT TO 16 PER CENT.** *'You can see more muscle,'* he exclaims. *'You can see my abs.'* Read more about John's success on page 156.

What you'll find so remarkable about this programme is how simple it is to follow, how often you'll eat – each meal and each snack is an easy, muscle-building, fat-burning treat – and how unlike any other 'diet' the Abs Diet is. Very simply, the Abs Diet is a plan that will ask you to:

▶ Eat three meals and three snacks each day, with each of your meals or snacks including several of the wide-ranging Powerfoods discussed in an upcoming chapter.

▶ Keep an eye out for a handful of diet busters that you'll learn to easily spot and cut down on – not eliminate.

▶ Perform a simple, 20-minute workout three times a week to turbocharge your fat loss and muscle growth.

The Abs Diet is so simple that, unlike most diets, we don't break it into phases, and we didn't design a complex 'maintenance' programme (just a few simple words of wisdom that you'll find on page 288). The weight loss and muscle gains are yours to keep for life, and so is the eating plan. We guarantee you won't be waiting for your 'diet' to end. You'll enjoy this programme so much – and be so wowed by the results – that you'll effortlessly follow this plan for life.

Other people have done it – other people who were in worse physical condition than you. When they talk about why it worked, they talk of the plan's simplicity and its ability to keep hunger in check. The Abs Diet is going to change your shape, your health, your life.

Chapter 6

SHOCKER: HOW LOW-CARB DIETS MAKE YOU FAT

The Truth about the Trend That's
Threatening Our Health

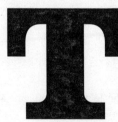**HROUGHOUT THIS BOOK, I'VE HIT**
you with scientific evi-
dence, persuaded you with
real-life testimonials, and
referenced study after study
to show how the Abs Diet works and why it makes sense
for anyone who wants to manage his weight and live a
healthy, active, disease-free life. But just for a moment, I
want to step away from all the hard science and take
you on a bit of a fantasy adventure. Come this way – I
promise you'll find it revealing.

First, I want you to imagine that you've taken a time machine back to the Middle Ages. You find yourself at the door of an alchemist's laboratory, where magic elixirs and potions fill the shelves and the echoes of mantras and spells fill the air. You've travelled long and hard, through terrifying dark woods and vast, arid deserts to seek out a Holy Grail of sorts: a concoction that legend says will make you lose weight, magically.

The sorcerer appears, and he holds up before you two vials. The first, he says, contains an elixir that will protect you from most of the diseases known to man. Its ingredients hold properties that will change your cholesterol profile and protect you from heart disease; help scour your body for toxins and protect you from the onslaught of cancer and the side effects of ageing; energize your body and your brain, making your thinking clearer and helping to immunize you from Alzheimer's; and, over the course of your long life, control your weight and keep obesity and diabetes at bay.

The second vial will do none of that. It will, in all likelihood, raise your cholesterol profile and increase your risk of cancer, stroke and heart disease, as well as other ailments. But, if you take it, it may help you lose weight dramatically – though only for a short period of time. And there's one more drawback: if you choose the second vial, you can never sip from the first.

Which do you choose?

In the past 5 years, millions of us have chosen vial number two.

Now, scrape the dust from the label on that vial and guess what it says? LOW-CARBOHYDRATE DIET.

The first vial, on the other hand, brims with all sorts of things: fruits and vegetables, wholegrain breads and cereals, beans and nuts – the sorts of thing that nature intended us to eat but diet plans like Atkins' do not. And over the long term, if we keep choosing vial number two, I think we're going to pay – heavily.

The Origins of a Sweet Tooth

TO UNDERSTAND WHY carbohydrates are important, we have to take another fantasy trip, this time back to the dawn of man. On the savannahs of Africa, the high plains of Europe, the wetlands of Asia and the woodlands and jungles of the Americas, primitive man learned how to feed himself from nature's banquet table. He learned how to fish and hunt, and later, how to domesticate animals and grow grain. But since he first stood upright, man has also had a craving for sweets.

As with all things, there's a reason why we crave sweets. The sweetest things on earth, back in those days before Mars bars, were fruits: wild berries, pears, citrus fruits and the like. Not coincidentally, fruits are also packed with nutrients: vitamins to fend off disease, minerals to assist with cell function and fibre to regulate hunger, control blood pressure and help ease digestion. Without our sweet tooth, we would have been happy to eat nothing but woolly mammoth and buffalo meat – the original Atkins programme. But nature saw to it that we craved the foods that would make us healthy.

Fast forward to today, when the sweetest things don't look anything like tangerines. Whereas our sweet tooth was once nature's way of protecting us from disease, now it's the food industry's way of tricking us into it. To satisfy our cravings, we turn to biscuits and cakes and chocolates instead of apples and pears and blackberries. That's one of the main reasons why so many people today are so fat. And it's one of the main reasons why, in the short-term, low-carb diets work.

By limiting carbohydrate intake, diets like Atkins create by-default weight loss. If you restrict yourself to just one class of foods – low-carb foods, in this instance – you're bound to lose weight. That's because the stuff you're used to munching on, from the doughnut you nosh in the car on the way to work to the Snickers bar you grab from the vending machine before your drive home, are now voided from your diet. You're eating less food, so you're taking in fewer calories, so you lose weight.

The other sneaky advantage of an Atkins diet is that it focuses on foods that are difficult to prepare and consume. It's easy to pop a bagel or a grapefruit into your briefcase; shove some steak and eggs in there instead, and things get a little messy. So low-carb diets restrict calories in two ways: by limiting food options, and by limiting the ease with which we can consume food.

But there are two major reasons why, in the long-term, low-carb diets won't work: Mother Nature and the almighty dollar.

Low-Carb Dilemma 1: Take That Out of Your Mouth!

SOMEONE WITH A SOUND understanding of nutrition and a sadistic streak could have a field day torturing low-carb enthusiasts. Here's an evil trick: take two pieces of soft, fresh, wholegrain bread. Slather one side with 2 tablespoons of natural peanut butter. Now take 75 g/2½ oz of blackberries, mash them lightly with a fork, and (this is where it gets really nasty) spread the mashed berries onto the other piece of bread. Put the two sides together and you've created the world's healthiest PB&J sandwich: 7 grams of fibre (over half what the average Briton gets in a single day), 25 per cent of your daily intake of vitamin C, 13 grams of protein, and *(sacre bleu!)* a forbidden 33 grams of carbohydrate. (Oh, by the way, it tastes incredible.)

Float this concoction in front of a low-carb enthusiast and you might as well be serving grilled rat entrails. (Come to think of it, they'd probably prefer the rat entrails. No carbs.) The sandwich is achingly sweet, soft and chewy, a delicious comfort food that, at the same time, is a cholesterol-busting nuclear missile. The fibre protects you from heart disease as well as from stroke and colon cancer. The vitamin C boosts your immune system. And the high-quality (meaning high in fibre) carbs give you long-burning energy and food for your brain. Yet phase one of the Atkins diet bans every single ingredient in this simple sandwich.

Every single one.

In fact, the Atkins diet focuses on something called *net carbs* that Atkins claims are the carbohydrates that actually affect blood sugar. A rough formula for working out net carbs is to subtract the number of fibre grams from the total number of carb grams. (The reasoning being that fibre doesn't affect blood sugar, spike insulin or contribute to fat storage.) By that calculation, this sandwich has about 33 net carbs. Phase one of the Atkins diet limits you to 20 net carbs *per day*. Eat this one super-good-for-you food, and *you'll have to fast for the next day and a half* to keep your Atkins diet in effect.

Maybe it's just me, but I think this whole low-carb plan is simply crackers. (Oh, sorry – not allowed to eat those.)

See, carbs are not our enemies. As I explained earlier, we crave carbs because we need them to protect us against a host of ailments. The low-carb craze works temporarily not because it limits carbs but because it limits food intake. And if I came out with some crazy diet plan that said you could only eat foods that are high in fat or low in protein or bigger than a breadbox or start with the letter P, believe me – you'd lose weight. For a little while, at least, until you couldn't look at pudding, parsnips and poultry ever again.

You'd lose weight because, by restricting your food intake, I've restricted your calorie intake. And the fact is, when you take in fewer calories than you burn, you lose weight; when you take in more calories than you burn, you gain weight. That's true regardless of where those calories come from. The Abs Diet works both by cutting the number of calories you take in through a sensible-but-satiating eating plan and by increasing the number of calories you burn away by improving your metabolic function. Fewer calories coming in here, a few more burned off there, and hey presto – weight loss. No magic, no deprivation and no pointing fingers at the evils of carbohydrates.

The confusion about carbs comes from the fact that in today's society, we're surrounded by high-carbohydrate foods that have had all their positive attributes stripped from them. Commercial bread baking seems to follow the rule that the whiter it gets, the less wholesome it becomes. The refined flours and sugars and sugar substitutes that you find in everything from biscuits to ice cream to mass-produced ketchup and peanut butter give us all the calories and none of the nutritional benefits of their original ancestors: whole grains and fruits. The lack of fibre in, say, a plain bagel causes the calories in the bagel to be digested quickly, flooding our bloodstreams with glucose, triggering spikes in the digestive hormone insulin – which then turns the blood sugar into fat cells and leaves us hungry once again.

But fruits, vegetables and wholegrain bread products have a very different effect on the body: they're digested slowly, giving us long-burning energy. Insulin levels stay steady while fibre scours our bodies for cholesterol and other harmful substances, and the vitamins and minerals inherent in those foods help protect us from a host of ills.

The longer we try to go without carbs, the more our bodies crave them. Eventually, you have to fall off a carb-restricting diet: your body is programmed to make you seek out carbs, just the way it's programmed to blink when something hurtles towards your eye. It's one of our natural defence mechanisms, and what Mother Nature wants, she will eventually get.

Then again, what the corporate world wants, it too will get. Which presents us with part two of why the low-carb craze is a disaster waiting to happen.

Low-Carb Dilemma 2: Follow the Money

REMEMBER WHAT I said about why the low-carb diet appears to work? Because it cuts out a majority of foods that people love to eat, and because it makes eating on the run difficult. Those two factors conspire to restrict calories, and fewer calories mean less weight.

Now, here's an easy question: how do food manufacturers make money? By selling you food. So what happens when millions of people decide they're going to stop buying all the confectionery bars, loaves of bread, packets of pasta and jars of sugary spreads that manufacturers have obligingly loaded with carbohydrates over the past half century?

Food manufacturers are going to have to come up with something else to sell. Something they can tout as low-carb, to appeal to Atkins-oriented dieters, but something that's familiar, easy to find, and even easier to consume. And so begins the next phase in the obesity epidemic.

In February 2004, the *New York Times* reported on the growing trend in America towards low-carb marketing among restaurants and grocery stores. Retailers were being advised by their business consultants to open up 'low-carb' aisles; restaurants were vying for the coveted 'Atkins approved' label to hang in their windows. And within 5 years, an estimated 728 new food products claiming to be low in carbohydrates hit the shelves. Today, you can snack on low-carb sweets, low-carb cake and low-carb brownies, washing it all down with a couple of bottles of low-carb beer.

To get a sneak preview of where all this is going, let's hop back into that time travel machine. This time, we're not going to the storied Middle Ages or the dawn of man . . . we're going back almost 20 years, to the beginnings of the last diet craze: the low-fat craze.

It's the early 1990s. The low-carb craze hasn't yet begun to blossom. (For better or worse, neither has Britney Spears.) But another mantra has begun to take hold: EAT LESS FAT.

This directive comes not from a book-peddling diet doc but from the government. Fat has been fingered as the root of all dietary evils: simply put, fatty foods translate into fatty people. Diet experts race to defend this idea, which on the face of it sounds pretty logical: dietary fat is more easily transformed into body fat, whereas carbohydrates are preferentially burned off for energy. Hence, swap your fat calories for carb calories and, voilà, you've entered into the magical weight-loss zone.

Quickly, food manufacturers move to capitalize on these exciting developments. As sales of skimmed milk rise, packages of reduced-fat, low-fat and fat-free cheeses, spreads, yogurts, ice creams, cakes and biscuits begin to fill the supermarket shelves. Some taste OK. Some taste like sugar-crusted cardboard. But what the hell – no fat, no foul. *Carbo-loading* becomes a byword of amateur athletes all across the country.

However, this whole low-fat theory comes with one big but. (Actually, it comes with millions of big butts, as the obesity rate

---

FIVE WAYS TO ADD MORE FIBRE

To your eggs: Half a chopped onion and a clove of garlic will add 1 gram of fibre to a couple of scrambled eggs.

To your sandwich: Hate wholemeal? Go with rye. Like wholemeal, it has 2 grams of fibre per slice. That's more than twice the amount of fibre in white.

To your dinner: Have a sweet potato. It has 2 grams more fibre than a typical white potato.

To your cereal: 75 g/2½ oz of raspberries adds 2 grams of fibre.

To your snack: Eat trail mix. 30 g/1 oz of Sultana Bran, 30 g/1 oz of mixed nuts and five dried apricot halves give you almost 7 grams of fibre.

has nearly tripled in the past 20 years.) Like today's low-carb craze, the low-fat craze originally appears to work because it creates a restrictive eating programme that eliminates certain foods and, hence, a certain number of calories. If you suddenly have to cut out countless steaks, baked goods, slabs of butter, nuts, dairy products and desserts, hey presto, you lose weight.

But, as with carbohydrates, our bodies crave fat. Fatty foods (beef, fish and dairy products, for instance) are usually high in muscle-building proteins and supply critical vitamins and minerals (the vitamin E in nuts and oils, the calcium in cheese and yogurt). So you can go on a low-fat diet for only so long before you wind up face-down in a carton of chocolate ice cream. That's the way Mother Nature planned it.

What she didn't plan for, however, was the craftiness of food marketers. Knowing that low-fat dieters are secretly pining for the old days when a nice slice of cake and a scoop of ice cream ended every celebratory meal, grocery manufacturers go into the laboratory and come out with hundreds of new low-fat foods. And that leads to what should go down in history as The Great Snack-Well's Debacle.

Nabisco conceives SnackWell's as the ultimate answer to the low-fat diet craze. SnackWell's, which you can still find on grocery shelves in America today, are fat-free and low-fat biscuits that somehow carry nearly all the flavour of full-fat biscuits. The secret is that Nabisco loads up the biscuits with extra sugar (except in the sugar-free varieties), so consumers can indulge their sweet tooth without ever missing the fat. How this development plays out in the mind of the average consumer is simple to predict:

'All I have to do to lose weight is to cut out fat.'

'Yo! These biscuits have no fat. Let's buy two packets!'

'Honey, did you eat that second packet of biscuits for breakfast? I wanted it!'

The magic bullet doesn't work, in part because we need to eat fats and in part because we've been fooled into thinking that we can eat whatever we want, in whatever quantity we want, as long as we aren't eating fat. So we scoff down sugar calories by the spoonful – and we all get just a little bit fatter in the process.

OK, hop out of the time machine – trip's over. It's a decade later and, instead of a low-fat craze, we're caught up in the throes of a low-carb craze. And the same scenario is playing out all over again. Every supermarket is filled with products – particularly 'meal replacement' bars – that are marketed with bywords like *low-carb* or *carb smart*.

Suddenly, it's not hard to eat low-carb any more. Today – and increasingly more so tomorrow – we can fill our shopping trolleys with all the foods we cut out for the past couple of years. Food marketers are altering the makeup of their products, packing them with soya protein and fibre and sugar alcohols – all ingredients that lower the 'net carb' impact of the food. Now, I'm all for more protein and fibre. Sugar alcohol, on the other hand, is nothing but empty calories that, in elevated quantities, cause gastric distress and flatulence – but hey, whatever turns you on.

What I am against is the notion that marketers are peddling that we can eat whatever and whenever we want, as long as we're not eating carbs. It is exactly the same trap we fell into 15 years ago: a restrictive diet that offers short-term success, turned into a food craze that guarantees even greater health risks and higher obesity rates.

And that's a time-travel destination no one wants to arrive at.

Chapter 7

THE ABS DIET NUTRITION PLAN

The Powerfoods and System
That Will Change Your Body

IN THE PREVIOUS CHAPTERS, I GAVE AN overview of some cool science – how your body reacts to different foods, why some fats are good and others are evil, and how some foods such as dairy products have a secret ingredient that helps your body burn fat. Science can be fun, but by this point in the book, you've probably got one burning question in your mind:

Hey, when can we eat?

So let's get right to it, because eating more of the right foods more often is the basis of the Abs Diet. Remember:

MORE FOOD = MORE MUSCLE = LESS FLAB

That's why the Abs Diet isn't a diet you'll feel you 'have to' stick to. It's one you'll want to stick to.

See, I've talked to lots of men who've tried diets, and many of them describe trying to stick to a strict diet plan as sort of like standing waist-deep in the ocean and being pummelled by one wave after another. Those waves come in the form of doughnuts the boss brought in, the office vending machine you're stuck with when the boss makes you work late, and the drinks to celebrate the firing of the boss who gave you all those doughnuts and late vending machine nights. When you're staring at a wave that's clearly bigger than you, you have three choices. You could run back to shore or try to jump over it, but those options will leave you with a suit full of sand. But if you dive through the wave head-on, you'll emerge unscathed. Same with a diet. You can try to run away by avoiding restaurants, parties, weddings and anywhere that's likely to tempt you with a big plate of chips. You can also try to take the high road, but ordering a salad and water after a football game hardly feels right. If you want a diet to work – if you want to emerge on the other side of this plan with a new body – your only choice is to have the flexibility and freedom to keep yourself from getting hungry and the knowledge that you can eat well no matter what.

You're about to dive into the Abs Diet.

Guideline 1: Eat Six Meals a Day

We're so used to hearing people talk about eating less food that it's become weight-loss doctrine. But as you remember from the physiology of metabolism, you have to eat more often to change your body composition. The new philosophy I want you to keep in mind is 'energy balance'.

Researchers at Georgia State University developed a technique to measure hourly energy balance – that is, how many calories you're burning versus how many calories you're taking in. The researchers found that if you keep your hourly surplus or deficit within 300 to 500 calories at all times, you will best be able to change your body composition by losing fat and adding lean muscle mass. Those subjects with the largest energy imbalances (those who were over 500 calories in either ingestion or expenditure) were the fattest, while those with the most balanced energy levels were the leanest. So if you eat only your three squares a day, you're creating terrific imbalances in your energy levels. Between meals, you're burning many more calories than you're taking in. At mealtimes, you're taking in many more than you're burning. Research shows that this kind of eating plan is great – if your dream is to be the next Michelin

OBESITY RISKS

Almost as important as what you eat is when you eat. Researchers at the University of Massachusetts analysed the eating habits of 500 men and women and found connections between the way people eat and the risk of becoming overweight.

HABIT	CHANGES YOUR RISK OF OBESITY BY
Eating at least one midday snack	–39 per cent
Eating dinner as your biggest meal of the day	+6 per cent
Waiting more than 3 hours after waking up to eat breakfast	+43 per cent
Eating more than a third of your meals in restaurants	+69 per cent
Going to bed hungry (3 or more hours after your last meal or snack)	+101 per cent
Eating breakfast away from home	+137 per cent
Not eating breakfast	+450 per cent

Man. But if you want to look slimmer, feel fitter and – not co-incidentally – live longer, then you need to eat more often. In the same study, subjects who added three snacks a day to three regular meals balanced out their energy better, lost fat and increased lean body mass (as well as increased their power and endurance).

In a similar study, researchers in Japan found that boxers who ate the same amount of calories a day from either two or six meals both lost an average of 5 kg/11 lb in 2 weeks. But the ones who ate six meals a day lost 1.4 kg/3 lb more fat and 1.4 kg/3 lb less muscle than the ones who ate only two meals.

There's science to support the fact that more meals work, but the plain-speak reason it works is because it does something that many diets don't do: it keeps you full and satiated, which will reduce the likelihood of a diet-destroying binge.

How it works: for scheduling purposes, alternate your larger meals with smaller snacks. Eat two of your snacks roughly 2 hours before lunch and dinner, and one snack roughly 2 hours after dinner.

Sample time schedule:

8 AM: breakfast

11 AM: snack

1 PM: lunch

4 PM: snack

6 PM: dinner

8 PM: snack

For a complete 7-day meal plan, check out page 120. It's not something you need to stick to religiously, just a suggestion for how you can make the Abs Diet work for you. It also shows how to incorporate the recipes you'll find in chapter 9 into your everyday life.

Guideline 2: Make These 12 Abs Diet Powerfoods the Staples of Your Diet

The Abs Diet will teach you to focus on (not restrict yourself to) a handful of food types – the Abs Diet Power 12 – to fulfil your core nutritional needs. These foods are all good for you. They're so good, in fact, that they'll just about single-handedly exchange your fat for muscle (provided you've kept your receipt). Just as important, I've designed the Power 12 to include literally thousands of food combinations. There are hundreds of dairy products, fruits and vegetables, lean meats and other choices to satisfy your tastes. Incorporating these Powerfoods into your six meals a day will satiate your tastes and cravings and keep you from feasting on the dangerous fat promoters in your diet.

You'll read more about these Powerfoods in chapter 8. For now, I just want you to remember:

Almonds and other nuts

Beans and pulses

Spinach and other green vegetables

Dairy (skimmed milk, fat-free or low-fat yogurt and cheese)

Instant hot oat cereal (unsweetened, unflavoured)

Eggs

Turkey and other lean meats

Peanut butter

Olive oil

Wholegrain breads and cereals

Extra-protein (whey) powder

Raspberries and other berries

12!

Guideline 3: Drink Smoothies Regularly

With schedules the way they are today, it's no wonder that your definition of a kitchen gadget is the one with a team logo that can open bottles. You need to make one exception for the kitchen gadget that won't fit on a key chain: the blender. I don't care how many speeds it has or how it looks, and I couldn't tell you the difference between a mince and a frappé. All I care about is how much stuff I can put in it and how good the stuff tastes when it comes out. (One thing I do recommend: get a blender with at least 400 watts, which will give it the power to handle chopping ice and shredding fruit and almost anything else you throw into it.)

When you consider that changing your body takes time, motivation and knowledge, consider your blender to be one of your most powerful tools in this plan. Smoothies made with a mixture of the Abs Diet Powerfoods can act as meal substitutions and as potent snacks, and they work for a few reasons:

▶ They require little time.

▶ Adding berries, flavoured whey powder or peanut butter will make them taste like dessert, which will satisfy your sweet cravings.

▶ Their thickness takes up a lot of space in your stomach.

I don't cook much. When I want a quick, healthy meal, I dump milk, low-fat vanilla yogurt, ice, uncooked instant oat cereal, natural peanut butter and a couple of teaspoons of chocolate whey powder into my blender and press a button. You can mix and match ingredients, depending on your tastes (see the recipes in chapter 9), but use the milk, yogurt, whey powder and ice as the base.

Here's the evidence showing these blended power drinks will help you control your weight:

▶ Researchers at Purdue University found that people stayed fuller longer when they drank thick drinks than when they drank thin ones – even when calories, temperatures and amounts were equal.

▶ A Penn State study found that men who drank yogurt shakes that had been blended until they doubled in volume ate 96 fewer calories a day than men who drank shakes of normal thickness.

▶ In a study presented at the North American Association of the Study of Obesity, researchers found that regularly drinking meal replacements increased a man's chance of losing weight and keeping it off for longer than a year.

▶ A University of Tennessee study found that men who added three servings of yogurt a day to their diets lost 61 per cent more body fat and 81 per cent more stomach fat over 12 weeks than men who didn't eat yogurt. Wow! Researchers speculated that the calcium helps the body burn fat and limit the amount of new fat your body can make.

How it works: drink a 240 ml/8 fl oz smoothie for breakfast, as a meal substitute or as a snack before or after your workout.

Guideline 4: Stop Counting

Though calorie burning is paramount to losing fat, calorie counting will make you lose focus and motivation. By eating these 12 Abs Diet Powerfoods and their many relatives, the foods themselves will, in a way, count your calories for you. They'll keep you healthy and feeling full and satisfied. Plus, the most energy-efficient foods are almost like doormen at a nightclub: they're not going to let any of the riffraff in without your approval.

Of course, that doesn't give you licence to speed down the

road of monstrous portions. Most of us claim that we watch what we eat, but most of us don't have a clue. A US Department of Agriculture study asked men what they ate, then checked it against reality. The truth: men aged 25 to 50 were eating twice the grains, fats and sweets that they estimated. If you eat six well-balanced meals, your body will regulate portions through things like fibre, protein, and the sheer volume of the smoothies. That said, it's always wise – especially at the beginning of the plan, when you're most vulnerable and adjusting to a new way of eating – to focus on portion control by limiting the servings of some foods, especially the ones with fat (like peanut butter) and carbohydrates (like rice or bread). A good rule: stick to one to two servings per food group, and keep the total contents of each

---

ABS DIET SUCCESS STORY

'I DEFLATED MY SPARE TYRE!'

Name: Patrick Austin

Age: 33

Height: 1.83 m/6'

Starting weight: 111 kg/17 st 7 lb

Six weeks later: 97.5 kg/15 st 5 lb

Patrick Austin thought he had the perfect solution for his spare tyre. At 1.83 m/ 6 ft and 111 kg/17 st 7 lb, and several years removed from school football, Austin had decided to take his fitness into his own hands. He hired a personal trainer and started to attack the fat.

But after 6 months of working one-on-one, nothing happened. 'I don't think the personal trainer personalized the programme for me,' Austin says. 'I think he used a general plan he used for everybody. There was no push.'

meal contained to the diameter of your plate. A height restriction is in effect.

Guideline 5:
Know What to Drink — And What Not To

I drink beer. I drink wine. I like to drink beer and wine, and gin and tonics on a hot summer day, and a lot of other things. There are health benefits to having one or two drinks a day, but there are many ways that alcohol can get you into trouble. Most important, alcohol — like cola and other soft drinks — adds calories that you don't need right now. These calories are empty calories because they don't actually help make you full or decrease the amount of

---

Then Austin stumbled across the Abs Diet and tried it. Within 10 days of his starting the Abs Diet, people in the gym were asking him what he'd been doing differently. He lost 6.8 kg/15 lb within the first couple of weeks, and he attributes it to a change in his approach to eating.

'I'm not the kind of person who eats a lot, but I was eating the wrong kinds of food,' Austin says. 'When I tried to lose weight before, I'd always watch my calories. But with the Abs Diet, you eat many meals — but concentrate on the right kinds of food.'

So instead of indulgences of cakes, pies and pastries after every meal, Austin downed smoothies, lean meats and eggs. 'Almonds became my best friend. They carry me over when I'm hungry in between meals.'

Austin also stayed dedicated to the workout — lifting weights 3 days a week and doing some type of cardio work on 3 other days.

Though he feels the best he's felt in years, Austin says he has one more goal. Every year, he and his wife go on a beach holiday with some other couples.

'I'm fanatical about the water. I love the pool. I love the beach. But I haven't gone shirtless on the beach in years. That's my goal this year,' Austin says. 'When we go this year, I'm going to be shirtless.'

food you'll eat. In fact, alcohol makes you eat more and encourages
your body to burn less fat. When Swiss researchers gave eight
healthy men enough alcohol to exceed their daily calorie requirements by 25 per cent (five beers for someone who eats 3,000 calories a day), they found that booze actually impaired men's ability
to burn fat by as much as 36 per cent. Booze also makes you store
fat. Your body sees alcohol as a poison and tries to get rid of it. So
your liver stops processing all other calories until it has dealt with
the alcohol. Anything else you eat while you're drinking most
likely will end up as fat. In some more indirect ways, alcohol can
inhibit your body's production of testosterone and human growth
hormone – two hormones that help burn fat and build muscle.

I hate to tell you to drink water, but drinking about eight
glasses a day has a lot of benefits. It helps keep you satiated (a lot
of times what we interpret as hunger is really thirst). Water
flushes the waste products your body makes when it breaks down
fat for energy or when it processes protein. You also need water to
transport nutrients to your muscles, to help digest food, and to
keep your metabolism ticking.

If you're serious about shedding stomach flab, I'd encourage
you to stay off the booze for the 6-week plan. At the least, limit
yourself to two or three alcoholic drinks per week. The best drinks
you can have are skimmed or semi-skimmed (low-fat) milk; water;
and green tea (or, if you must, a can of diet drink a day).

Guideline 6: For One Meal a Week, Forget the First Five Guidelines

I would never advocate cheating on your spouse, your employer or
your taxes. But I want you to cheat on this diet. I want you to take
one meal during the week and forget everything about good carbohydrates and good fats. Have half a pizza, a burger, or whatever

it is that you miss the most while you're on this plan. Have it, savour it, and then dig back in for another week. I want you to cheat for a couple of reasons. One, I want you to control when you cheat. Plan your cheat meal for the week – whether it's Saturday night out, during a football game, or whenever. But if you keep it planned, you'll stick to it. The way to control your cravings is to satisfy them every once in a while. If you can make it through 6 days, you reward yourself and know that 6 days of good eating is a regime you can stick to over the long term.

And there's another important reason I want you to cheat: because it'll actually help you change your body. A successful diet plan is about how you eat most of the time, not how you eat all of the time. In fact, a high-calorie day of eating can rev up your metabolism. Researchers at the American National Institutes of Health found that men who ate twice as many calories in a day as they normally did increased their metabolism by 9 per cent in the 24-hour period that followed. But here's where you have to show control. I think that this diet plan allows you to have plenty of foods that are both good and good for you, but I know you will crave other foods that don't fit into our guidelines. Think of this cheat meal as the carrot at the end of a good week of eating. I encourage you to enjoy your meal of gluttony and, please, don't make the carrot literally a carrot.

THE 7-DAY ABS DIET MEAL PLAN

Unlike most diet plans, which are laden with complex, hard-to-follow rules and forbidden foods you love but have to live without, the Abs Diet lets you eat the foods you love, keeps your cravings at bay and helps you control stress – all at the same time. Here's an example of how you can structure a week of eating. It's not written in stone, by any means: mix up the meals. Substitute whenever you want. Heck, I don't care if you eat the same thing every day for a week. The purpose of this chart is simply to show you how to follow the principles of the Abs Diet. So enjoy!

MONDAY

Breakfast: One tall glass (240 to 350 ml/8 to 12 fl oz) Abs Diet Ultimate Power Smoothie (page 152); make extra for later

Snack 1: 2 teaspoons peanut butter, raw vegetables (as much as you want)

Lunch: Turkey or roast beef sandwich on wholegrain bread, 240 ml/8 fl oz skimmed milk, 1 apple

Snack 2: 30 g/1 oz almonds, 200 g/7 oz berries

Dinner: Mas Macho Meatballs (page 161)

Snack 3: 240 to 350 ml/8 to 12 fl oz Abs Diet Ultimate Power Smoothie

TUESDAY

Breakfast: Eggs Beneficial Sandwich (page 155)

Snack 1: 2 teaspoons peanut butter, 1 bowl hot oat cereal or high-fibre cereal

Lunch: The I-Am-Not-Eating-Salad Salad (page 158)

Snack 2: 3 thin slices turkey breast, 1 large orange

Dinner: Bodacious Brazilian Chicken (page 161)

Snack 3: 30 g/1 oz almonds, 115 g/4 oz cantaloupe melon

WEDNESDAY

Breakfast: One tall glass (240 to 350 ml/8 to 12 fl oz) Strawberry Field Marshall Smoothie (page 153); make extra for later

Snack 1: 30 g/1 oz almonds, 30 g/1 oz raisins

Lunch: Guac and Roll (page 158)

Snack 2: 1 stick string cheese, raw vegetables (as much as you want)

Dinner: Chilli-Peppered Steak (page 162)

Snack 3: 240 to 350 ml/8 to 12 fl oz Strawberry Field Marshall Smoothie

THURSDAY

Breakfast: 1 slice wholegrain bread with 1 tablespoon peanut butter, 1 medium orange, 75 g/2½ oz All-Bran cereal with 240 ml/8 fl oz skimmed milk, 145 g/5 oz berries

Snack 1: 240 ml/8 fl oz low-fat yogurt, 1 can V8 juice

Lunch: Guilt-Free BLT (page 158)

Snack 2: 3 thin slices roast beef, 1 large orange

Dinner: Philadelphia Fryers (page 162)

Snack 3: 2 teaspoons peanut butter, 240 ml/8 fl oz low-fat ice cream

FRIDAY

Breakfast: One tall glass (240 to 350 ml/8 to 12 fl oz) Banana Split Smoothie (page 153); make extra for later

Snack 1: 30 g/1 oz almonds, 115 g/4 oz cantaloupe melon

Lunch: Hot Tuna (page 159)

Snack 2: 3 thin slices roast beef, 1 large orange

Dinner: Chilli Con Turkey (page 162)

Snack 3: 240 to 350 ml/8 to 12 fl oz Banana Split Smoothie

SATURDAY

Breakfast: One tall glass (240 to 350 ml/8 to 12 fl oz) Halle Berries Smoothie (page 153); make extra for later

Snack 1: 1 bowl high-fibre cereal, 240 ml/8 fl oz low-fat yogurt

Lunch: Leftover Chilli Con Turkey

Snack 2: 2 teaspoons peanut butter, 1 or 2 slices wholegrain bread

Dinner: *Cheat meal!* Have whatever you've been craving this week: beer and a burger, beer and pizza, beer and sausages – anything you can dream of.

Snack 3: 240 to 350 ml/8 to 12 fl oz Halle Berries Smoothie

SUNDAY

Breakfast: The I-Haven't-Had-My-Coffee-Yet Sandwich (page 156)

Snack 1: 2 teaspoons peanut butter, 1 can V8 juice

Brunch (relax – it's Sunday): 2 scrambled eggs, 2 slices wholegrain toast, 1 banana, 240 ml/8 fl oz skimmed milk

Snack 2: 3 thin slices roast beef, 1 slice reduced-fat cheese

Dinner: BBQ King (page 164)

Snack 3: 30 g/1 oz almonds, 240 ml/8 fl oz low-fat ice cream

Chapter 8

THE ABS DIET POWER 12

Meet the Powerfoods That Will Shrink Your Gut and Keep You Healthy for Life

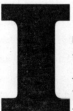N THE PREVIOUS CHAPTER, I GAVE YOU the six guidelines for following the Abs Diet and touched briefly on the Abs Diet Power 12. Now, I want you to meet each of these 12 superheroes up close.

These 12 foods make up a large part of your diet. The more of these foods you eat, the better your body will be able to increase lean muscle mass and avoid storing fat. Though you can base entire meals and snacks around these foods, you don't have to. But do follow these guidelines.

► Incorporate two or three of these foods into each of your three major meals and at least one of them into each of your three snacks.

▶ Diversify your food at every meal to get
a combination of protein, carbohydrates and fat.

▶ Make sure you sneak a little bit of protein
into each snack.

How to read the key For at-a-glance scanning, I've included the
following icons under the descriptions of each of the Abs Diet Powerfoods. Each icon demonstrates which important roles each food
can help play in maintaining optimum health.

Builds muscle: foods rich in muscle-building plant and
animal proteins qualify for this seal of approval, as do
foods rich in certain minerals linked to proper muscle maintenance, such as magnesium.

Helps promote weight loss: foods high in calcium and
fibre (both of which protect against obesity) as well as
foods that help build fat-busting muscle tissue earn this badge of
respect.

Strengthens bone: calcium and vitamin D are the most
important bone builders, and they protect the body against
osteoporosis. But beware: high levels of sodium can leach calcium
out of bone tissue. Fortunately, all of the Powerfoods are naturally
low in sodium.

Lowers blood pressure: any food that's not high in
sodium can help lower blood pressure – and score this des-
ignation – if it has beneficial amounts of potassium, magnesium
or calcium.

Fights cancer: research has shown that there is a lower
risk of some types of cancer among those people who maintain low-fat, high-fibre diets. You can also help foil cancer by
eating foods that are high in calcium, beta-carotene or vitamin C.
In addition, all cruciferous (cabbage-type) and allium (onion-type)
vegetables get the cancer protection symbol because research has
shown they help prevent certain kinds of cancer.

Improves immune function: vitamins A, E, B$_6$ and C; folic acid; and the mineral zinc help to increase the body's immunity to certain types of disease. This icon indicates a Power-food with high levels of one or more of these nutrients.

Fights heart disease: artery-clogging cholesterol can lead to trouble if you eat foods that are predominant in saturated and trans fats, while foods that are high in mono-unsaturated or polyunsaturated fats will actually help protect your heart by keeping your cholesterol levels in check.

1: Almonds and Other Nuts

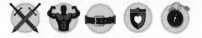

Superpowers: builds muscle, fights cravings

Secret weapons: protein, monounsaturated fats, vitamin E, fibre, magnesium, folic acid (peanuts), phosphorus

Fights against: obesity, heart disease, muscle loss, wrinkles, cancer, high blood pressure

Sidekicks: pumpkin seeds, sunflower seeds, avocados

Imposters: salted or smoked nuts

These days, you hear about good fats and bad fats the way you hear about good cops and bad cops. One's on your side, and one's gonna beat you silly. Biscuits fall into the latter category, but nuts are clearly out to help you. They contain the monounsaturated fats that clear your arteries and help you feel full.

All nuts are high in protein and monounsaturated fat. But almonds are like Jack Nicholson in *One Flew over the Cuckoo's Nest*: they're the king of the nuts. A handful of almonds provides half the amount of vitamin E you need in a day and 8 per cent of the calcium. They also contain 19 per cent of your daily require-ment of magnesium – a key component for muscle building. In a Western Washington University study, people taking extra magnesium were able to lift 20 per cent more weight and build more muscle than those who weren't. Eat as much as two handfuls of almonds a day. A Toronto University study found that men can eat this amount daily without gaining any extra weight. A Purdue University study showed that people who ate nuts high in mono-unsaturated fat felt full an hour and a half longer than those who ate fat-free food (rice cakes, in this instance). If you eat 60 g/2 oz of almonds (about 24 of them), it should be enough to suppress your appetite – especially if you wash them down with 240 ml/8 fl oz of water. The fluid helps expand the fibre in the nuts to help you feel fuller. Also, try to keep the nuts' nutrient-rich skins on them.

Here are ways to seamlessly introduce almonds or other nuts into your diet.

▶ Add chopped nuts to plain peanut butter.

▶ Toss a handful on cereal, yogurt or ice cream.

▶ Put slivers in an omelette.

▶ For a quick popcorn alternative: spray a handful of almonds with olive oil cooking spray and bake at 200°C/400°F/gas 6 for 5 to 10 minutes. Take them out of the oven, and sprinkle them with a mixture of either brown sugar and cinnamon, or cayenne pepper and thyme.

One caveat, before you get all nutty: smoked and salted nuts don't make the cut here, because of their high sodium content. High sodium can mean high blood pressure.

2: Beans and Pulses

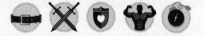

Superpowers: builds muscle, helps burn fat, regulates digestion

Secret weapons: fibre, protein, iron, folic acid

Fights against: obesity, colon cancer, heart disease, high blood pressure

Sidekicks: lentils, peas, bean dips, hummus, edamame (green soya beans)

Imposters: refried beans, which are high in saturated fats; baked beans,
 which are high in sugar

Most of us can trace our resistance to beans to some unfortunately
timed intestinal upheaval (third-year maths class, a first date
gone awry). But beans are, as the song says, good for your heart;
the more you eat them, the more you'll be able to control your
hunger. Black, haricot, lima (butter), kidney, chickpea – you pick
the bean (as long as it's not refried – refried beans are loaded with
fat). Beans are a low-calorie food packed with protein, fibre and
iron – ingredients crucial for building muscle and losing weight.
Gastrointestinal disadvantages notwithstanding, they serve as
one of the key members of the Abs Diet cabinet because of all their
nutritional power. In fact, you can swap in a bean-heavy dish for a
meat-heavy dish a couple of times per week; you'll be lopping a lot
of saturated fat out of your diet and replacing it with higher
amounts of fibre.

The best beans for your diet are:

▶ Soya beans

▶ Haricot beans

▶ Chickpeas

▶ Black beans

▶ Cannellini beans

▶ Kidney beans

▶ Lima (butter) beans

3: Spinach and Other Green Vegetables

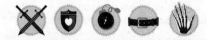

Superpowers: neutralizes free radicals, which are molecules that
 accelerate the ageing process

Secret weapons: vitamins including A, C and K; folic acid; minerals
  including calcium and magnesium; fibre; beta-carotene

Fights against: cancer, heart disease, stroke, obesity, osteoporosis

Sidekicks: cruciferous vegetables like broccoli, cabbage and brussels
  sprouts; green, yellow, red and orange vegetables like asparagus,
  peppers and fresh beans

Imposters: none, as long as you don't fry them or smother them in fatty
  cheeses

You know vegetables are packed with important nutrients, but
they're also a critical part of your body-changing diet. I like
spinach in particular because one serving supplies nearly a full
day's worth of vitamin A and half of your vitamin C. It's also
loaded with folic acid – a vitamin that protects against heart disease, stroke and colon cancer. To incorporate it, you can take the

LEAN GREEN MACHINES

Essentially, iceberg lettuce is the nutritional equivalent of a plastic office plant
– it adds a little colour, but mostly it just takes up space. Iceberg may be
cheap and plentiful, but it contains almost no fibre, vitamins or minerals. If
you're going to eat salad, you might as well eat salad with some *cojones* to it.
Check out this green dream team.

The cancer killer: romaine (Cos) lettuce. This celery-flavoured green is one
of the best vegetable sources of beta-carotene – 712 micrograms per head.
A University of Illinois study showed that high levels of beta-carotene inhibited
the growth of prostate cancer cells by 50 per cent.

The bone builder: rocket. 30 g/1 oz of these mustard-flavoured leaves has 15
per cent of the bone-building mineral calcium found in a glass of whole milk
and 100 per cent less saturated fat. There's also some magnesium in every
bite, for even more protection against osteoporosis.

The pipe protector: watercress. It's a pepper-flavoured HEPA filter for your
body. Watercress contains phytochemicals that may prevent cigarette smoke
and other airborne pollutants from causing lung cancer.

The heart healer: endive. It's slightly bitter and a little crisp, and it offers
twice the fibre of iceberg lettuce. A head of endive also provides almost 20

fresh stuff and use it as lettuce on a sandwich, or try stir-frying it with a little garlic and olive oil.

Another potent power vegetable is broccoli. It's high in fibre and more densely packed with vitamins and minerals than almost any other food. For instance, it contains nearly 90 per cent of the vitamin C of fresh orange juice and almost half as much calcium as milk. It is also a powerful defender against diseases like cancer because it increases the enzymes that help detoxify carcinogens. *Tip:* with broccoli, you can skip the stalks. The florets have three times as much beta-carotene as the stems, and they're also a great source of other antioxidants.

If you hate vegetables, you can learn to hide them but still reap the benefits. Try puréeing them and adding them to pasta sauce or chilli. The more you chop and purée vegetables, the more

per cent of your daily requirement of folic acid. People who don't get enough of this essential B vitamin may have a 50 per cent greater risk of developing heart disease.

The brain booster: mustard greens. These spicy, crunchy greens are packed with the amino acid tyrosine. In a recent US military study, researchers found that eating a tyrosine-rich meal an hour before taking a test helped soldiers significantly improve both their memories and their concentration.

The anti-ageing agent: pak choi (bok choy). Think of it as a cabbage-flavoured multivitamin. A bowl of pak choi has 23 per cent of your daily requirement of vitamin A and a third of your vitamin C, along with three tongue-twisting, cancer-fighting, age-reducing phytochemicals: flavonoids, isothiocyanates and dithiolthione.

The sight sharpener: spinach. Spinach is a top source of lutein and zeaxanthin, two powerful antioxidants that protect your vision from the ravages of old age. A Tufts University study found that frequent spinach eaters had a 43 per cent lower risk of age-related macular degeneration.

The pressure punisher: kohlrabi. Kohlrabi tastes like the love child from a tryst between a cabbage and a turnip. Each serving contains around 15 per cent of your daily requirement of potassium (to help keep a lid on your blood pressure), along with glucosinolate, a phytochemical that may prevent some cancers.

invisible they become and the easier it is for your body to absorb them. With broccoli, sauté it in garlic and olive oil, and douse it with a hot sauce.

4: Dairy (Skimmed Milk, Fat-Free or Low-Fat Yogurt and Cheese)

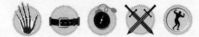

Superpowers: builds strong bones, fires up weight loss

Secret weapons: calcium, vitamins A and B_{12}, riboflavin, phosphorus, potassium

Fights against: osteoporosis, obesity, high blood pressure, cancer

Sidekicks: none

Imposters: whole milk, frozen yogurt

Dairy is nutrition's version of a typecast actor. It gets so much attention for one thing it does well – strengthening bones – that it gets little or no attention for all the other stuff it does well. It's about time for dairy to accept a breakout role as a vehicle for weight loss. Just take a look at the mounting evidence: a University of Tennessee study found that dieters who consumed between 1,200 and 1,300 milligrams of calcium a day lost nearly twice as much weight as dieters getting less calcium. In a Purdue University study of 54 people, those who took in 1,000 milligrams of calcium a day (about 700 ml/1¼ pints of fat-free milk) gained less weight over 2 years than those with low-calcium diets. Researchers think that calcium probably prevents weight gain by increasing the breakdown of body fat and hampering its formation. Low-fat yogurt, cheeses and other dairy products can play an important role in your diet. But as your major source of calcium, I recommend milk for one primary reason: volume. Liquids can take up valuable room in your stomach and send the signal to your brain that you're full. Adding in a sprinkle of chocolate powder can also help curb sweet cravings while still providing nutritional power.

5: Instant Hot Oat Cereal (Unsweetened, Unflavoured)

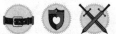

Superpowers: boosts energy and sex drive, reduces cholesterol, maintains blood sugar levels

Secret weapons: complex carbohydrates and fibre

Fights against: heart disease, diabetes, colon cancer, obesity

Sidekicks: high-fibre cereals like All-Bran

Imposters: cereals with added sugar, glucose syrup and corn syrup

Oats are the Bo Derek of your larder: a perfect 10. You can eat oats at breakfast to propel you through sluggish mornings, a couple of hours before a workout to feel fully energized by the time you hit the weights, or at night to avoid a late-night binge. I recommend instant oats for their convenience. But I want you to buy the unsweetened, unflavoured variety and use other Powerfoods such as milk and berries to enhance the taste. Preflavoured oat cereal often comes loaded with sugar calories.

Oatmeal contains soluble fibre, meaning that it attracts fluid and stays in your stomach longer than insoluble fibre (like vegetables). Soluble fibre is thought to reduce blood cholesterol by binding with digestive acids made from cholesterol and sending them out of your body. When this happens, your liver has to pull cholesterol from your blood to make more digestive acids, and your bad cholesterol levels drop.

Trust me: you need more fibre, both soluble and insoluble. Doctors recommend we get at least 18 to 20 grams of fibre per day, but most of us get half that. Fibre is like a bouncer for your body, kicking out troublemakers and showing them the door. It protects you from heart disease. It protects you from colon cancer by sweeping carcinogens out of the intestines quickly.

A Penn State study also showed that oatmeal sustains your blood sugar levels longer than many other foods, which keeps your insulin levels stable and ensures you won't be ravenous for the few hours that follow. That's good, because spikes in the production of insulin slow your metabolism and send a signal to the body that it's time to start storing fat. Since oatmeal breaks down slowly in the stomach, it causes less of a spike in insulin levels than foods like bagels. Include it in a smoothie or as your breakfast. (A US Navy study showed that simply eating breakfast raised metabolism by 10 per cent.)

Another cool fact about oatmeal: preliminary studies indicate that oatmeal raises the levels of free testosterone in your body, enhancing your body's ability to build muscle and burn fat and boosting your sex drive.

6: Eggs

Superpowers: builds muscle, burns fat

Secret weapons: protein, vitamin B_{12}, vitamin A

Fights against: obesity

Sidekicks: none

Imposters: none

For a long time, eggs were considered pure evil, and doctors were more likely to recommend tossing eggs at passing cars than into omelette pans. That's because just two eggs contain enough cholesterol to put you over your daily recommended value. Though you can cut out some of the cholesterol by removing part of the yolk and using the whites, more and more research shows that eating an egg or two a day will not raise your cholesterol levels, as once previously believed. In fact, we've learned that most blood cholesterol is made by the body from dietary fat, not dietary cholesterol. And that's why you should take advantage of eggs and their powerful makeup of protein.

The protein found in eggs has the highest 'biological value' of protein – a measure of how well it supports your body's protein need – of any food. In other words, the protein in eggs is more effective in building muscle than protein from other sources, even milk and beef. Eggs also contain vitamin B_{12}, which is necessary for fat breakdown.

7: Turkey and Other Lean Meats (Lean Steak, Chicken, Fish)

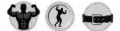

Superpowers: builds muscle, improves the immune system

Secret weapons: protein, iron, zinc, creatine (beef), omega-3 fatty acids (fish), vitamins B_6 (chicken and fish) and B_{12}, phosphorus, potassium

Fights against: obesity, various diseases

Sidekicks: shellfish, lean (back) bacon

Imposters: sausage, streaky bacon, cured meats, ham, fatty cuts of steak like T-bone and rib-eye

A classic muscle-building nutrient, protein is the base of any solid diet plan. A 2008 US study found that people who ate higher amounts of protein were more likely to stick to their diets for one year than those who ate more carbohydrates instead. The researchers say it is because protein is more satiating than carbs are, so the people who ate more meat and fish weren't as hungry as the people on the high-carb diet. You already know that it takes more energy for your body to digest the protein in meat than it does to digest carbohydrates or fat, so the more protein you eat, the more calories you burn. Many studies support the notion that high-protein diets promote weight loss. In one study, researchers in Denmark found that men who substituted protein for 20 per cent of their carbs were able to increase their metabolism and increase the number of calories they burned every day by up to 5 per cent.

Among meats, turkey is a rare bird. Turkey breast is one of the leanest meats you'll find, and it packs nearly one-third of your daily requirements of niacin and vitamin B_6. Dark meat, if you prefer, has lots of zinc and iron. One caution, though: if you're roasting a whole turkey for a family feast, avoid self-basting birds, which have been injected with fat.

Beef is another classic muscle-building protein. It's the top food source for creatine – the substance your body uses when you lift weights. Beef does have a downside; it contains saturated fats, but some cuts have more than others. Look for topside, rump or fillet steak; sirloins are less fatty than prime ribs and T-bones. Wash down that steak with a glass of skimmed milk. Research shows that calcium (that magic bullet again!) may reduce the amount of saturated fat your body absorbs. Cuts on the left side of the chart contain less fat but still pack high amounts of protein.

LEAN BEEF (55 calories and 2–3 grams of fat per 30-g/1-oz serving)	MEDIUM-FAT BEEF (75 calories and 4–5 grams of fat per 30-g/1-oz serving)
Skirt (flank) steak	Chuck steak
Minced beef (extra-lean or lean)	Minced beef (not labelled lean or extra-lean)
Roast beef	Corned beef
Fillet	

To cut down on saturated fats even more, concentrate on fish like tuna and salmon, because they contain a healthy dose of

Fat Content of Meat
(115 g/4 oz, raw, without skin or bone)

	TOTAL (G)	SATURATED (G)
Skinless chicken breast	1.41	0.37
Veal steak	2.45	0.74
Wild rabbit	2.63	0.78
Lean minced beef	4	1.50
Cured ham	4.68	1.56
Duck breast	7.4	2.3
Chicken drumstick	5.05	1.34
Lean pork fillet (tenderloin)	5.06	1.79
Beef, sirloin steak	5.15	2
Turkey leg	7.62	2.34
Turkey breast	7.96	2.17
Beef, topside	8.02	3
Fillet steak	8.02	3
Lean pork chop	8.19	2.85
Porterhouse steak	8.58	3
Lean minced turkey	9.37	2.55
Veal breast	9.73	3.80
Rib-eye steak	18.03	7.30
T-bone steak	19.63	7.69
Ham	21.40	7.42
Pork belly	60.11	21.92
Cured pork	91.29	33.32

omega-3 fatty acids as well as protein. Those fatty acids lower levels of a hormone called leptin in your body. Several recent studies suggest that leptin directly influences your metabolism: the higher your leptin levels, the more readily your body stores calories as fat. Researchers at the University of Wisconsin found that mice with low leptin levels have faster metabolisms and are able to burn fat faster than animals with higher leptin levels. Mayo Clinic researchers studying the diets of two African tribes found that the tribe that ate fish frequently had leptin levels nearly five times lower than the tribe that primarily ate vegetables. A bonus benefit: researchers in Stockholm studied the diets of more than 6,000 men and found that those who ate no fish had three times the risk of prostate cancer than those who ate it regularly. It's the omega-3s that inhibit prostate cancer growth.

Whether you eat fish or not, I want you to consider adding ground flaxseed to your food. As I pointed out earlier, 1 tablespoon contains only 60 calories, but it packs in omega-3 fatty acids and has nearly 4 grams of fibre. It has a nutty flavour, so you can sprinkle it into a lot of different recipes, add some to your meat or beans, spoon it over cereal or add a tablespoon to a smoothie.

8: Peanut Butter (Natural, Sugar-Free)

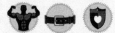

Superpowers: boosts testosterone, builds muscle, burns fat

Secret weapons: protein, monounsaturated fat, vitamin E, niacin, magnesium

Fights against: obesity, muscle loss, wrinkles, cardiovascular disease

Sidekicks: cashew and almond butters

Imposters: mass-produced sugary and trans fatty peanut butters

Yes, PB has its disadvantages: it's high in calories, and it doesn't go down well when you order it in restaurants. But it's packed with those heart-healthy monounsaturated fats that can increase your body's production of testosterone, which can help your muscles grow and your fat melt. In one 18-month experiment, people who integrated peanut butter into their diet maintained weight loss better than those on low-fat plans. A recent study from the University of Illinois showed that diners who had monounsaturated fats before a meal (in this case, it was olive oil) ate 25 per cent fewer calories during that meal than those who didn't.

Practically speaking, PB also works because it's a quick and versatile snack – and it tastes good. Since a diet that includes an indulgence like peanut butter doesn't leave you feeling deprived, it's easier to follow and won't make you fall prey to other cravings. Use it on an apple, on the go, or to add flavour to potentially bland smoothies. Two caveats: you can't gorge on it because of its fat content; limit yourself to about 3 tablespoons per day. And you should look for all-natural peanut butter, not the mass-produced brands that have added sugar.

9: Olive Oil

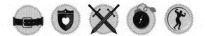

Superpowers: lowers cholesterol and boosts the immune system

Secret weapons: monounsaturated fat, vitamin E

Fights against: obesity, cancer, heart disease, high blood pressure

Sidekicks: rapeseed (canola) oil, peanut oil, sesame oil

Imposters: vegetable and hydrogenated vegetable oils, trans fatty acids, margarine

You read extensive information on the value of high-quality fats like olive oil in chapter 3. But it's worth reiterating here: olive oil and its brethren will help you eat less by controlling your food cravings; they'll also help you burn fat and keep your cholesterol in check. Do you need any more reason to pass the bottle?

10: Wholegrain Breads and Cereals

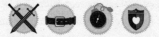

Superpower: prevents your body from storing fat

Secret weapons: fibre, protein, thiamin, riboflavin, niacin, pyridoxine, vitamin E, magnesium, zinc, potassium, iron, calcium

Fights against: obesity, cancer, high blood pressure, heart disease

Sidekicks: brown rice, wholewheat pasta

Imposters: processed bakery products like white bread, bagels, doughnuts

There's only so long a person can survive on an all-protein diet or an all-salad diet or an all-anything diet. You will crave carbohydrates because your body needs carbohydrates. The key is to eat the ones that have been the least processed – carbs that still have all their heart-healthy, belly-busting fibre intact.

Grains like wheat, corn, oats, barley and rye are seeds that come from grasses, and they're broken into three parts – the germ, the bran and the endosperm. Think of a kernel of corn. The biggest part of the kernel – the part that blows up when you make popcorn – is the endosperm. Nutritionally it's pretty much a big dud. It contains starch, a little protein and some B vitamins. The germ is the smallest part of the grain; in the corn kernel, it's that little white seedlike thing. But while it's small, it packs the most nutritional power. It contains protein, oils and the B vitamins thiamin, riboflavin, niacin and pyridoxine. It also has vitamin E and the minerals magnesium, zinc, potassium and iron. The bran is the third part of the grain and the part where all the fibre is stored. It's a coating around the endosperm that contains B vitamins, zinc, calcium, potassium, magnesium and other minerals.

So what's the point of this little biology lesson? Well, get this: when food manufacturers process and refine grains, guess which two parts get tossed out? Yup, the bran, where all the fibre and minerals are, and the germ, where all the protein and vitamins are. And what they keep – the nutritionally bankrupt endosperm (that is, starch) – gets made into pasta, bagels, white bread, white rice, and just about every other wheat product and baked good you'll find. Crazy, right? But if you eat products made with all the parts of the grain – wholegrain bread, pasta, brown rice – you get all the nutrition that food manufacturers are otherwise trying to cheat you out of.

Wholegrain carbohydrates can play an important role in a healthy lifestyle. In an 11-year study of 16,000 middle-aged people, researchers at the University of Minnesota found that consuming three daily servings of whole grains can reduce a person's mortality risk over the course of a decade by 23 per cent. (Tell that to your mate who's eating low-carb.) A 2008 study at the University of Nottingham found that eating a breakfast of whole grains and fresh fruit will help you burn 50 per cent more fat during a workout than you would after eating a breakfast of refined carbs. That's because when we eat refined carbs (like bagels or sugary cereals) blood sugar spikes and muscles store more glycogen, which the body uses instead of fat for fuel. Wholegrain bread, by contrast, keeps insulin levels low, which helps muscles store less glycogen so your body can stoke its engine with fat. In this diet, wholegrain bread is especially versatile because it'll supplement any kind of meal with little prep time. Toast for breakfast, sandwiches for lunch, with a dab of peanut butter for a snack. Don't believe the hype. Carbs – the right kind of carbs – are good for you.

Warning: food manufacturers are very sneaky. Sometimes, after refining away all the vitamins, fibre and minerals from wheat, they'll claim to 'put back the goodness' by adding wheat-germ. It's a trick! Truly nutritious breads and other products will say WHOLEMEAL or WHOLEGRAIN. Don't be fooled.

11: Extra-Protein (Whey) Powder

Superpowers: builds muscle, burns fat

Secret weapons: protein, cysteine, glutathione

Fights against: obesity

Sidekick: ricotta cheese

Imposter: soya protein

Protein powder? What the heck is that? It's the only Abs Diet Powerfood that you may not be able to find at the supermarket, but it's the one that's worth the trip to a health food store. I'm talking about powdered whey protein, a type of animal protein that packs a muscle-building wallop. If you add whey powder to your meal – in a smoothie, for instance – you may very well have created the most powerful fat-burning meal possible. Whey protein is a high-quality protein that contains essential amino acids that build muscle and burn fat. But it's especially effective because it has the highest amount of protein for the fewest number of calories, making it fat's kryptonite. Smoothies with some whey powder can be most effective before a workout. A 2001 study at the University of Texas found that weightlifters who drank a shake containing amino acids and carbohydrates before working out increased their protein synthesis (their ability to build muscle) more than weightlifters who drank the same shake after exercising. Since exercise increases bloodflow to tissues, the theory goes that having whey protein in your system when you work out may lead to a greater uptake of amino acids – the building blocks of muscle – in your muscle.

But that's not all. Whey protein can help protect your body from prostate cancer. Whey is a good source of cysteine, which your body uses to build a prostate cancer–fighting antioxidant called glutathione. Adding just a small amount may increase glutathione levels in your body by up to 60 per cent.

By the way, the one great source of whey protein in your supermarket is ricotta cheese. Unlike other cheeses, which are made from milk curd, ricotta is made from whey – a good reason to visit your local Italian restaurant.

HOW TO PICK PRODUCE

A lot of us grew up with an aversion to fruits and vegetables, mostly caused by doting mums who boiled greens into a pulp and then insisted that by not eating them, we were somehow responsible for kids in Asia not having enough to eat. Today, you've got two ways to prove your mum wrong: first, by showing her how really delicious fresh produce can be, if you know how to pick it and prepare it, and second, by showing her a picture of a sumo wrestler. (Hey, somebody was getting enough food.)

Berries. Before you buy raspberries or strawberries, flip the carton over. You're looking for nature's expiry date: juice stains. You want berries you can eat without looking like you've been fingerprinted.

Corn on the cob. The sweetest ears are slightly immature, with kernels that don't go all the way to the end of the cob. Toss 'em, husks and all, onto a medium-hot grill. Cook for 10 minutes, then peel back all but the last layer of husk. Grill 5 more minutes for that just-smoked flavour.

Watermelon. Forget colour, shape or size: watermelons are best judged by weight. The heavier a melon is, the more water it contains, and water is what helps give a melon its flavour.

Cantaloupe. Don't knock on a melon to check its ripeness; slap it instead. You're listening for a hollow ring, not a dull thud or an inhuman scream.

Tomatoes. Look for tomatoes that are firm and heavy for their size. They should have a sweet tomato aroma. If you generally don't like tomatoes, try the yellow kind; they tend to have a sweeter, less acidic flavour than red varieties.

Peaches. Look for well-coloured fruit with no green spots. The flesh should yield slightly when lightly pressed and should have a fragrant aroma. (Fragrant like a peach, not fragrant like your cousin Freddy.)

12: Raspberries and Other Berries

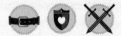

Superpowers: protects your heart; enhances eyesight; improves balance, coordination and short-term memory; prevents cravings

Secret weapons: antioxidants, fibre, vitamin C, tannins (cranberries)

Fights against: heart disease, cancer, obesity

Sidekicks: most other fruits, especially apples and grapefruit

Imposters: jellies, most of which eliminate fibre and add sugar

Depending on your taste, any berry will do. I like raspberries as much for their power as for their taste. They carry powerful levels of antioxidants, all-purpose compounds that help your body fight heart disease and cancer; the berries' flavonoids may also help your eyesight, balance, coordination and short-term memory. A bowl (145 g/5 oz) of raspberries packs 4 grams of fibre and more than 100% of your daily requirement of vitamin C.

Blueberries are also loaded with the soluble fibre that, like oatmeal, keeps you fuller longer. In fact, they're one of the most healthy foods you can eat. Blueberries beat 39 other fruits and vegetables in the antioxidant power ratings. (One study also found that rats that ate blueberries were more coordinated and smarter than rats that didn't.)

Strawberries contain another valuable form of fibre called pectin (as do grapefruits, peaches, apples and oranges). In a study from the *Journal of the American College of Nutrition*, subjects drank plain orange juice or juice spiked with pectin. The people who got the loaded juice felt fuller after drinking it than those who got the juice without the pectin. The difference lasted for an impressive 4 hours.

SPECIAL REPORT

YOUR WEIGHT IS NOT YOUR FAULT

The Sneaky Ways Food Manufacturers
Are Scheming to Make You Fat

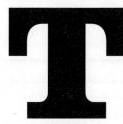**HE SIX NUTRITIONAL GUIDELINES** of the Abs Diet and the ABS DIET POWER 12 will steer you down the street of good eating. Follow those principles, and you will soon see remarkable changes in your appearance and your health. Now, I can take you down the street and show you the roads that lead you to a life of more muscle and less fat, but I'd be one shoddy tour guide if I didn't warn you of the two biggest hoodlums lurking around the corner. They're the two ingredients that will sneak up on you and rob you of

all of the progress you've made on the diet: high-fructose corn syrup (HFCS) and trans fat. Luckily, thanks to the work of some scientific sketch artists, we have a pretty good idea of how they operate and when they strike.

And they strike often. These two new calorie bombs were hardly ever eaten before the mid-1970s, but now they're lurking in all sorts of foods, especially in the US. No wonder a recent study by the Centers for Disease Control and Prevention found that in 1971, American men averaged a daily intake of 2,450 calories and that women ate an average of 1,542, but in the year 2000, American men were averaging about 2,618 calories (up 7 per cent), while women were eating 1,877 calories (up 22 per cent). Did we all get hungrier? No. The food got supersized.

Now remember: this diet isn't about restriction or deprivation, so I'm not going to tell you to turn away and run every time you see HFCS or trans fats. What I do want you to do is get to know them. Know what foods they come in, and understand how they can destroy all the good things you've done to change your body. See, one of the secrets to the success of the Abs Diet is that it incorporates ways to deal with this terrible twosome. By eating six balanced meals and snacks with ingredients that increase your metabolism, you'll have less of a craving for foods that contain the bad substances. And by allowing yourself one cheat meal per week, you can schedule a place where you indulge in some of your favourite foods that fall into the criminal category. Instead of resisting them all the time, give them an occasional wave, but know that it's in your best interest not to make too many trips to this side of town.

High-Fructose Corn Syrup

HFCS is a man-made sweetener that's cheaper and sweeter than sugar. Food manufacturers love it because it enhances their profits, so they are adding it to more and more foods. Cereal. Ketchup.

Fizzy drinks. Pasta sauce. Biscuits. Even some meal replacement bars, which are supposed to be good for you, may well contain HFCS.

We're talking about a processed sweetener that didn't even exist in the food chain until the 1970s. And HFCS is really, really, really bad for you. That's because it's packed with calories, but your body doesn't recognize these calories. In fact, HFCS shuts off your body's natural appetite control switches, so you can eat and eat and eat far beyond what your body would normally be able to handle. You probably know guys who can down a 2-litre bottle of Coke in a single sitting. Well, guess what? Before HFCS was invented, humans couldn't do that. Our natural appetite control switches would kick in, detect the sugar we were consuming, and say *'No more!'* But by shutting off the switches that control appetite, HFCS – a true junk food – is making us fat. In 1970, for example, Americans ate about 225g/ 8 oz of HFCS per person per year. By the late 1990s, every person was consuming about 28 kg/62 lb every year. That's 228 additional calories per person per day.

The problem with HFCS is not the corn syrup; it's the fructose – a sugar that occurs naturally in fruit and honey. Corn syrup is primarily made of glucose, which can be burned as a source of immediate energy, stored in your liver or muscles for later use or, as a last resort, turned to fat. But corn syrup isn't as sweet as other sugars, which is why HFCS became so popular. It's cheap and doubly sweet.

Unlike glucose, your body doesn't use fructose as an immediate source of energy; it metabolizes it into fat. While the small amount of fructose you get naturally through fruit and honey won't make you fat, eating HFCS is sort of like setting up an IV that pumps fat directly to your gut. Some of the worst offenders are fizzy drinks: consumption has increased enormously in the last few decades. So the amount of HFCS we're getting is unprecedented – and many researchers think there's a direct link between the huge amount of HFCS we're consuming and the huge numbers we're seeing on the scales.

Go back to what you know about carbohydrates. When you eat any carbohydrate – whether it contains glucose or starch – your body releases insulin to regulate your body weight. First, it tries to push the carbs into your muscle cells to be used as energy and facilitates carb storage in the liver for later use. Then it suppresses your appetite, telling your body that you've had enough. Finally, it stimulates production of another protein, leptin, which is manufactured in your fat cells. In essence, leptin helps regulate how much fat you store and helps increase your metabolism to keep your weight in check. Like the mother-in-law who tries to tell you how to raise your kids, fructose screws up a system that was working perfectly fine without it. Fructose doesn't stimulate insulin and therefore doesn't increase the production of leptin – and that's the most important argument against fructose and HFCS: without insulin and leptin, your body has no shut-off mechanism. You can drink 4 litres of Coke or down two cartons of frozen yogurt, and your body thinks you haven't eaten since the last time Bill Gates borrowed money from his dad.

Soft drinks are one of the main sources of HFCS, but researchers tried to determine whether the drinks themselves or HFCS was the problem. The verdict: HFCS. In a study in the *American Journal of Clinical Nutrition*, researchers took two groups of overweight people and had one group drink regular soft drinks while the other group drank diet versions (which contain no HFCS) for 10 weeks. The group given regular soft drinks gained weight and increased their body fat, as well as saw an increase in their blood pressure. The diet drinks group consumed fewer calories than they normally would, lost weight, reduced body fat and lowered blood pressure.

Even if you don't drink fizzy drinks, HFCS can still sneak up on you. Here's where nutritional labels come in handy. If a label says 'sugar' or 'cane sugar', the product contains sucrose, which is a 50/50 blend of glucose and fructose. That doesn't seem to be much of a problem. If HFCS is listed first or second, look at the chart on the nutrition label to see how much sugar the food contains. If it's just a gram or two, don't get in a sweat about it. But if you see a food that has 8 or more grams of sugar and HFCS is prominent on the list of ingredients, do what you do when you get turned down for a date: move along to something else. The body can deal with a little of anything, but when your HFCS numbers start looking like Freddy Flintoff's batting figures, that's when you're headed for trouble. Consult the substitution chart for low-maintenance fixes.

FOODS POTENTIALLY HIGH IN HFCS OR FRUCTOSE	REPLACE WITH
Regular soft drinks	Unsweetened sparkling water or diet drinks
Commercial sweets (like jelly beans)	Chocolate (check the label; some chocolate bars have HFCS)
Pancake syrup	Real maple syrup
Frozen yogurt	Ice cream
Fruit-flavoured yogurt	Organic yogurt
Highly sweetened cereals	Sugar-free or low-sugar cereals
Pasta sauce	Sugar-free pasta sauce
Energy bars	HFCS-free energy bars

Trans Fats

I touched on trans fats in chapter 4, but they're so bad for you that I want to revisit them here. Used in thousands of common prepared foods, from frozen waffles to biscuits, french fries to bran muffins, trans fats are simply vegetable oil infused with hydrogen.

Trans fats are difficult to digest, so they increase the amount of bad cholesterol in your blood and can dramatically boost your risk of heart disease, weaken your immune system, and even cause diabetes. Scientists estimate that trans fats contribute to numerous premature deaths every year.

In the 1950s, scientists first made the link between saturated fat, cholesterol and heart disease. After the discovery, manufacturers scrambled to find a way to cut saturated fats. Their solution was a process called partial hydrogenation, in which vegetable oil is combined with hydrogen and heated to extremely high temperatures. As the molecules in the oil warm up, they bond with the hydrogen, transforming a liquid to a solid. Voilà, trans fatty acid. Immediately, it was a hit. Restaurants liked it because they could fill their fryer vats with it and keep it hot without smoking

SUBSTITUTE TEACHING

Partially hydrogenated oils are everywhere. You can't eliminate them from your diet, but if you pick the right brands of the foods you love, you can dramatically reduce the amount you're taking in on a daily basis.

IF YOU WANT	PICK THIS TRANS FAT–FREE OPTION
Chocolate	Green & Black's chocolate
Cheese spread	Cheez Whiz Light (a number of other reduced-fat ones are OK too – check the label)
Biscuits	Pure butter shortbread (some gingernuts, oatcakes and digestive biscuits are OK too – check the label)
Corn chips	Tyrells vegetable chips
Crackers	Ryvita or Finn Crisp rye crackers
French fries	McCain Oven Chips
Frozen waffles	Kellogg's Special K fat-free waffles
Margarine	I Can't Believe It's Not Butter Spread or Bertolli olive oil spread
Potato crisps	Ruffles Natural sea-salted, reduced-fat crisps

up their kitchens. Trans fatty acid was cheaper than butter and lasted longer, so restaurants could buy it in bulk without worrying about it spoiling. It soon became the staple of what you find in those two sinful supermarket aisles – crisps and biscuits.

Since trans fat doesn't exist in nature, your body has a much harder time processing it than it does other types of fats. If your body were a railway line, the first stop trans fat would make would be at your heart. Trans fat increases your bad cholesterol and lowers your good cholesterol, and it increases blood levels of a compound called lipoprotein. The more lipoprotein you have in your system, the greater your risk of developing heart disease. Researchers have even found that trans fat could increase your risk of cancer.

After years of struggling with the food industry (which didn't want to list trans fat, for fear that consumers' knowing about it would result in the loss of billions of dollars every year), the US Food and Drug Administration passed a regulation in mid-2003 that forced companies to list trans fat on food labels. But companies were free to phase in the change over several years. The UK Food & Drink Federation says that UK food manufacturers have been reducing levels in their products, but at the moment they are under no obligation to list the amount they include. In the meantime, here are some things you can do to limit the amount of trans fat in your diet.

AT THE SUPERMARKET	AT HOME	AT A RESTAURANT
Check the ingredients list for HYDROGENATED or PARTIALLY HYDROGENATED. The higher these ingredients are on the label, the more trans fats they contain (with the exception of peanut butter, which contains trace amounts).	Pick high-protein breakfasts like eggs or lean (back) bacon instead of waffles. If you have toast, use peanut butter instead of margarine.	Ask what kind of oil the chef uses. You want to hear olive oil.

AT THE SUPERMARKET	AT HOME	AT A RESTAURANT
Decode the food label. Add all the fat grams together that are listed on the label, and then subtract that number from the total fat content. The number you're left with is the estimate for the amount of trans fat in the food.	Snack on baked crisps (potato chips) or crisps fried in olive oil rather than other fats.	Order foods that are baked or grilled – not fried.
Buy margarine that is free of trans fat, like Bertolli. Check the label.	Flavour vegetables or baked potatoes with olive oil, sesame oil, or even butter-flavoured spray instead of margarine.	Avoid garlic bread, which may be filled with trans fat. It's better to pick a baked potato, soup or salad.
Translate the labels. Cholesterol-free doesn't mean it's free of trans fat. Only fat-free means that.	Make a sandwich with a tortilla wrap or a pitta instead of bread.	Blot oil from your chips/fries as quickly as possible. A napkin can absorb excess grease.

Partially hydrogenated oils are in thousands of foods. You can't eliminate them entirely, but most experts recommend cutting as many grams of trans fat as you can from your diet. Here's how some popular foods stack up.

FOOD	TRANS FAT (g)
1 Cornish pasty	5
1 order of nachos with cheese	5
1 large order of fries	3
2 biscuits	2
15 g/½ oz hard margarine	2
1 small cinema popcorn	2
1 slice of apple pie (shop bought)	2
1 waffle	1

Chapter 9

THE ABS DIET MEAL PLAN

Using Powerfoods in Quick and Easy Recipes

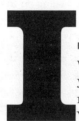**F YOU'RE LIKE A LOT OF THE GUYS I WORK** with and a lot of the guys I know, you spend more time in the bathroom than you do in the kitchen. You simply don't have time to cook. You grab breakfast on your way out, fill up on coffee when you get to work, eat lunch with colleagues or clients, and swing by the vending machine at 4. By the time you get home at 8, 9, or 10 o'clock, there are only two things you feel like doing – and both of them happen in your bed.

Look, I'm exactly the same way. I don't have the time, energy, or creative impulse to cook. My hob is more likely to be littered with bills and junk mail than pots and pans, and my oven is more likely to be used for storage

than for cooking. (Once, my mum came for a visit and acciden-
tally baked my basketball.) The first time I cooked dinner for
my girlfriend, she accurately identified the meal as 'some kind
of meat'.

So what you're going to see on the next few pages has been
extensively idiot-proofed, and if you can operate a blender and a
frying pan, you can handle these meals.

Most of these recipes are ones you can make quickly – some in
less than 5 minutes. I also know that you're not going to make
every meal, so I've included sample combinations of foods that
make properly balanced meals, utilizing the Powerfoods. For the
dinners, servings sizes are larger than one, so you can also use
the leftovers for lunch.

Abs Diet Smoothies

Smoothies are one of the best parts about being on the Abs Diet.
They take less than 3 minutes to make. They pack in multiple
high-nutrient foods. They fill you up. If that's not enough, they
can also taste like a five-star dessert. You can come up with your
own concoctions by using skimmed milk, low-fat vanilla yogurt,
whey powder and ice as the main ingredients. Oatmeal and fruit
make nice additions, as does a spoonful of peanut butter. Include
all ingredients in a blender, and blend until smooth. For extra
volume, add more ice. Here are some examples.

Abs Diet Ultimate Power Smoothie (number of Powerfoods: 5)

240 ml/8 fl oz skimmed milk

2 tablespoons low-fat vanilla yogurt

50 g/1¾ oz instant hot oat cereal (dry
   weight), nuked in water

2 teaspoons peanut butter

2 teaspoons chocolate whey powder

6 ice cubes, crushed

Makes 2 240-ml/8-fl oz servings

*Per serving: 250 calories/1045 kJ; Protein 12 g; Carbs 34 g; Fat 7 g;
Saturated fat 1 g; Sodium 158 mg; Fibre 2.5 g*

Strawberry Field Marshall Smoothie (number of Powerfoods: 5)

120 ml/4 fl oz low-fat vanilla yogurt

240 ml/8 fl oz skimmed milk

2 teaspoons peanut butter

170 g/6 oz frozen strawberries

2 teaspoons whey powder

6 ice cubes, crushed

Makes 2 240-ml/8-fl oz servings

Per serving: 202 calories/845 kJ; Protein 11 g; Carbs 27 g; Fat 6 g; Saturated fat 2 g; Sodium 177 mg; Fibre 1.5 g

Cereal Killer (number of Powerfoods: 4)

40 g/1½ oz All-Bran cereal

240 ml/8 fl oz skimmed milk

60 g/2 oz blueberries

1 tablespoon honey

2 teaspoons whey powder

6 ice cubes, crushed

Makes 2 240-ml/8-fl oz servings

Per serving: 148 calories/619 kJ; Protein 9 g; Carbs 28 g; Fat 1 g; Saturated fat 0 g; Sodium 276 mg; Fibre 6 g

Banana Split Smoothie (number of Powerfoods: 3)

1 banana

120 ml/4 fl oz low-fat vanilla yogurt

2 tablespoons frozen orange juice concentrate

240 ml/8 fl oz skimmed milk

2 teaspoons whey powder

6 ice cubes, crushed

Makes 2 240-ml/8-fl oz servings

Per serving: 181 calories/757 kJ; Protein 9 g; Carbs 36 g; Fat 1 g; Saturated fat 0.5 g; Sodium 139 mg; Fibre 1 g

Halle Berries Smoothie (number of Powerfoods: 4)

50 g/1¾ oz instant hot oat cereal (dry weight), nuked in water or skimmed milk

180 ml/6 fl oz skimmed milk

100 g/3½ oz mixed frozen blueberries,

strawberries and raspberries

2 teaspoons whey powder

3 ice cubes, crushed

Makes 2 240-ml/8-fl oz servings

Per serving: 154 calories/647 kJ; Protein 8 g; Carbs 27 g; Fat 2 g; Saturated fat 0.5 g; Sodium 83 mg; Fibre 3 g

PB&J Smoothie (number of Powerfoods: 5)

180 ml/6 fl oz low-fat vanilla yogurt

180 ml/6 fl oz skimmed milk

2 teaspoons peanut butter

1 medium banana

90 g/3 oz frozen strawberries

2 teaspoons whey powder

4 ice cubes, crushed

Makes 2 240-ml/8-fl oz servings

*Per serving: 267 calories/1117 kJ; Protein 12 g; Carbs 42 g; Fat 6 g;
Saturated fat 2 g; Sodium 179 mg; Fibre 2 g*

Summer Smoothie (number of Powerfoods: 4)

115 g/4 oz frozen strawberries

1 banana

1 wedge honeydew melon

120 ml/4 fl oz low-fat vanilla yogurt

180 ml/6 fl oz skimmed milk

2 teaspoons vanilla whey powder

3 ice cubes, crushed

Makes 2 240-ml/8-fl oz servings

*Per serving: 200 calories/836 kJ; Protein 9 g; Carbs 41 g; Fat 1 g;
Saturated fat 0.5 g; Sodium 147 mg; Fibre 2 g*

Abs Diet Breakfasts

Between getting a shower, skimming the paper and the last-minute gluing you need to do on your kid's science project, breakfast is the martyr meal of the day. You usually sacrifice it for anything else that needs your attention. But if you had to rank the six meals in order of importance, the first meal would rank first. Breakfast wakes up your metabolism and tells it to start burning fat, decreasing your risk of obesity. The quickest way to incorporate the Abs Diet into your breakfast is to combine potent foods (the Powerfoods) to make meals, such as:

▶ 240-ml/8-fl oz smoothie

▶ 2 tablespoons of peanut butter on wholegrain toast and 2 slices of back bacon

▶ 2 Shredded Wheat with 240 ml/8 fl oz skimmed milk, 3 turkey sausages and 75 g/2½ oz of berries

▶ 2 scrambled eggs, 2 slices of wholegrain toast, 1 banana and 240 ml/8 fl oz of skimmed milk

▶ 30 g/1 oz of high-fibre cereal mixed with 15 g/ ½ oz of Crunchy Nut Cornflakes, 2 tablespoons of almonds and 180 ml/6 fl oz skimmed milk

▶ 1 slice of wholegrain bread with 1 tablespoon of peanut butter, 1 medium orange, 40 g/1¼ oz of All-Bran cereal with 120 ml/4 fl oz skimmed milk, and 75 g/2½ oz berries

On the weekends or on mornings when you can spare a few more minutes, these breakfasts will also deliver the appropriate nutritional punch.

Eggs Beneficial Sandwich (number of Powerfoods: 5)

1 large whole egg	1 slice back bacon, grilled
3 large egg whites	1 tomato, sliced, or 1 green pepper
1 teaspoon ground flaxseed	(capsicum), sliced
2 slices wholemeal bread, toasted	120 ml/4 fl oz orange juice

1. Scramble the whole egg and egg whites in a bowl. Add the ground flaxseed.

2. Fry in a nonstick pan spritzed with vegetable oil spray, and dump onto the toast.

3. Add bacon and tomatoes, peppers, or other vegetables of your choice. Drink the juice.

Makes 1 serving

Per serving: 400 calories/1672 kJ; Protein 30 g; Carbs 39 g; Fat 14 g; Saturated fat 4 g; Sodium 1164 mg; Fibre 5 g

Breakfast Bacon Burger (number of Powerfoods: 4)

1 wholemeal muffin

½ teaspoon trans fat–free spread

1 egg

1 low-fat cheese slice

1 slice back bacon, grilled

Vegetables of choice

1. Split the muffin, toast it, and add the spread.

2. Break the egg in a microwavable dish, prick the yolk with a cocktail stick, and cover the dish with cling film.

3. Microwave on high for 30 seconds. Let stand for 30 seconds. Add the cheese, egg and bacon to the muffin, then nuke for 20 seconds.

4. Add vegetables to taste.

Makes 1 serving

Per serving: 350 calories/1463 kJ; Protein 25 g; Carbs 26 g; Fat 17 g; Saturated fat 6 g; Sodium 1023 mg; Fibre 3 g

The I-Haven't-Had-My-Coffee-Yet Sandwich (number of Powerfoods: 3)

1½ teaspoons low-fat cream cheese

1 wholemeal pitta, halved to make 2 pockets

2 slices turkey or ham

Lettuce or green vegetable

ABS DIET SUCCESS STORY

'I TURNED FLAB INTO MUSCLE!'

Name: John Betson

Age: 25

Height: 1.77 m/5'10"

Starting weight: 81.7 kg/12 st 12 lb

Six weeks later: 74.9/11 st 11 lb

Fathers pass down a lot of things to their sons, but John Betson inherited one thing from his dad that he didn't want: flabby breast tissue. 'I've always had flab on my chest and, since I was a kid, I've had to work hard to keep from looking like the Dolly Parton of the gym,' Betson says.

At school, football took care of it, but after graduation a 60-hour-a-week desk job added roundness in two places he didn't want – his gut and his pecs. Realizing he was 6.8 kg/15 lb overweight, Betson decided to get back in shape. 'I wanted to make sure I looked good for my wife,' he says. 'I didn't want to give her a reason to look elsewhere.'

1. Spread the cream cheese in the pockets of the pitta.

2. Stuff with the meat and vegetables.

3. Put in mouth. Chew and swallow.

Makes 1 serving

Per serving: 260 calories/1086 kJ; Protein 15 grams; Carbs 45 g; Fat 3 g; Saturated fat 1 g; Sodium 410 mg; Fibre 3 g

Abs Diet Lunches

In the middle of a workday, a burger bar or pizza joint can be more tempting than that colleague with the great glutes. Be strong! You can still follow the eating plan no matter where you are. Grilled chicken or chilli and a baked potato are usually good options. In sit-down situations, you can also order smartly. Some good combinations include a salad with grilled chicken or salmon, vegetables, almonds or other nuts, and a sprinkling of balsamic vinegar and olive oil. You can also order a piece of lean meat –

The first week on the Abs Diet was the toughest because it was so counter-intuitive. Betson was used to eating only two meals a day. He'd eat a banana and a packet of crackers for lunch. Then, armed with the feeling that he hadn't eaten much during the day, he'd load up on massive helpings of meat loaf and pizza for dinner. But the Abs Diet required him to eat often – up to six times a day. 'I felt fat at first because I was eating so much, but after the first week, I loved it. I loved the food, and I loved feeling stronger and more energetic,' he says.

He also lifted weights 3 days a week and did cardio work 3 days a week, which resulted in a dramatic change in body composition. He lost 6.8 kg /15 lb and decreased his percentage of body fat from 23 to 16 per cent. 'You can see more muscle. You can see my abs,' he says.

What's even more amazing is that at the same time Betson started the Abs Diet, he quit smoking – a time when most people gain weight.

Down from a 91-cm/36-in waist to an 81- or 84-cm/32- or 33-in waist, Betson says the biggest change he's felt is actually internal. He says, 'Confidence – having more confidence – is the biggest improvement I've seen.'

either on wholegrain bread or by itself – with a serving of vege-tables. Ask for salsa or a small dish of olive oil for dipping. If you bring your lunch or eat it at home, these are some other options.

The I-Am-Not-Eating-Salad Salad (number of Powerfoods: 4)

60 g/2 oz grilled chicken

1 head romaine (Cos) lettuce

1 tomato, chopped

1 small green pepper (capsicum), chopped

1 medium carrot, chopped

3 tablespoons virtually fat-free Italian dressing or 1 teaspoon olive oil

1 tablespoon grated Parmesan cheese

1 tablespoon ground flaxseed

1. Chop the chicken into small pieces.

2. Mix all the ingredients together, and store in the fridge. Eat on multigrain bread or by itself.

Makes 1 serving

Per serving: 350 calories/1463 kJ; Protein 28 g; Carbs 14 g; Fat 20 g; Saturated fat 6 g; Sodium 250 mg; Fibre 6 g

Guilt-Free BLT (number of Powerfoods: 3)

¾ tablespoon reduced-fat mayonnaise

1 wholemeal tortilla

2 slices turkey bacon, cooked

60 g/2 oz roasted turkey breast, diced

2 slices tomato

2 leaves lettuce

1. Smear the mayo on the tortilla.

2. Line the middle of the tortilla with the bacon and top with the turkey breast, tomato and lettuce.

3. Roll it tightly into a tube.

Makes 1 serving

Per serving: 330 calories/1379 kJ; Protein 32 g; Carbs 10 g; Fat 19 g; Saturated fat 5 g; Sodium 168 mg; Fibre 1 g

Guac and Roll (number of Powerfoods: 4)

170 g/6 oz oil-packed tuna

150 ml/5 fl oz guacamole

2 tomatoes, chopped

1 teaspoon lemon juice

1 tablespoon reduced-fat mayonnaise

1 teaspoon ground flaxseed

2 15-cm/6-inch wholemeal rolls

1. Combine the first six ingredients in a bowl and blend thoroughly with a fork.

2. Split the rolls in half, and fill each half with a quarter of the mixture.

Makes 2 servings

Per serving: 622 calories/2599 kJ; Protein 35 g; Carbs 58 g; Fat 29 g; Saturated fat 5 g; Sodium 818 mg; Fibre 9 g

Hot Tuna (number of Powerfoods: 4)

2 sticks celery, chopped

1 onion, chopped

60 g/2 oz reduced-fat mozzarella cheese, grated

90 g/3 oz reduced-fat cottage cheese

170 g/6 oz brine-packed tuna, drained and flaked

4 tablespoons reduced-fat mayonnaise

1 tablespoon lemon juice

3 wholemeal muffins, split in half

1. Preheat your oven to 180°C/350°F/gas 4. In a nonstick frying pan over a low heat, cook the celery and onion until softened. Add the cheeses, tuna, mayo and lemon juice, and cook the mixture just long enough to warm it through.

2. Spread one-sixth of the mixture on each muffin half. Put the muffin halves on a baking sheet, and bake for 10 minutes.

Makes 2 servings

Per serving: 768 calories/3210 kJ; Protein 44 g; Carbs 81 g; Fat 32 g; Saturated fat 8 g; Sodium 1,300 mg; Fibre 10 g

Yo Soup for You (number of Powerfoods: 3)

225 g/8 oz chicken breast

225 g/8 oz chopped onion

1 teaspoon olive oil

2 cloves garlic, finely chopped

1.5 litres/2½ pints low-sodium chicken stock

145 g/5 oz canned haricot or cannellini beans, drained

60 g/2 oz carrots, finely chopped

115 g/4 oz sweetcorn

100 g/3½ oz canned peeled tomatoes

2 tablespoons chopped basil or parsley

¼ teaspoon ground black pepper

1. In a large saucepan over a low heat, cook the chicken and onion in the oil for about 10 minutes, or until the onion is golden brown. Add the garlic and cook for 1 minute.

2. Add the stock, beans and carrots. Bring to the boil. Add the sweetcorn and tomatoes (with their juice). Cook for 15 minutes. Add the herbs and pepper.

Makes 4 servings

Per serving: 176 calories/735 kJ; Protein 18 g; Carbs 20 g; Fat 4 g; Saturated fat 1 g; Sodium 571 mg; Fibre 4 g

Hurry Curry (number of Powerfoods: 3)

120 ml/4 fl oz fat-free natural yogurt

120 ml/4 fl oz reduced-fat mayonnaise

3 tablespoons finely chopped onions

1 teaspoon grated fresh ginger

1 teaspoon curry powder

455 g/1 lb boneless, skinless chicken
breast, cut into 1-cm/½-in strips

1 teaspoon paprika

½ teaspoon ground black pepper

150 g/5½ oz brown rice, cooked

1. In a small bowl, mix the yogurt, mayonnaise, onion, ginger and curry powder.

2. Place the chicken in a medium bowl. Sprinkle with the paprika and pepper. Toss until coated.

3. In a nonstick frying pan over a medium heat, cook the chicken for 4 to 5 minutes. Stir in the yogurt mixture. Cook, stirring, for 2 minutes. Serve over rice.

Makes 2 servings

Per serving: 700 calories/2940 kJ; Protein 60 g; Carbs 70 g; Fat 25 g; Saturated fat 6 g; Sodium 359 mg; Fibre 2 g

Nice-to-Meat-You Sandwich (number of Powerfoods: 3)

2 slices wholemeal bread

60 g/2 oz sliced roast beef

2 inner leaves romaine (Cos) lettuce

1 teaspoon reduced-fat mayonnaise

30 g/1 oz low-fat Cheddar cheese

1. Stack everything up into a sandwich.

Makes 1 serving

Per serving: 347 calories/1450 kJ; Protein 34 g; Carbs 25 g; Fat 13 g; Saturated fat 5 g; Sodium 1154 mg; Fibre 4 g

Ragin' Cajun (number of Powerfoods: 2)

100 g/3½ oz brown rice

115 g/4 oz canned black beans

1 teaspoon Benecol spread

Dash of Tabasco

1. Cook the rice according to the packet instructions.

2. Add the beans (with their liquid), spread and Tabasco. Stir. Refrigerate overnight and nuke at lunch.

Makes 1 serving

Per serving: 315 calories/1317 kJ; Protein 13 g; Carbs 55 g; Fat 6 g; Saturated fat 1 g; Sodium 333 mg; Fibre 5 g

Abs Diet Dinners

Dinner is the place where most of us wind down and pork up. That's because we spend the day serving others. By dinnertime, we're hungry to have some of our own demands met. On this plan, you'll have already fuelled up four times before dinner, so you'll feel pleasantly hungry, not ravenous. These meals give you the taste of sin – without the actual guilt.

Mas Macho Meatballs (number of Powerfoods: 3)

455 g/1 lb extra-lean minced beef

45 g/1½ oz breadcrumbs

1 large onion, diced

1 clove garlic, finely chopped

1 tablespoon ground flaxseed
   or whey powder

1 jar (480 ml/16 fl oz) tomato sauce
   (passata)

4 wholemeal rolls

60 g/2 oz reduced-fat mozzarella
   cheese, grated

1. Mix the beef, breadcrumbs, onion, garlic and flaxseed or whey powder into golf ball-sized meatballs.

2. In a nonstick frying pan over a medium heat, cook the meatballs until browned all over. Drain the fat from the pan, and add the tomato sauce.

3. While the mixture is warming, use a fork to scoop out some of the bread in the rolls to form shallow trenches. Spoon the meatballs and sauce into each trench, sprinkle with grated mozzarella, and top with the top half of the roll.

Makes 4 servings

Per serving: 391 calories/1634 kJ; Protein 35 g; Carbs 45 g; Fat 10 g; Saturated fat 4 g; Sodium 1,340 mg; Fibre 6 g

Bodacious Brazilian Chicken (number of Powerfoods: 2)

1 lemon

1 lime

1 tablespoon ground flaxseed

240 ml/8 fl oz tomato sauce (passata)

180 ml/6 fl oz frozen orange juice
   concentrate

2 cloves garlic, finely chopped

1 teaspoon dried Italian seasoning

4 boneless, skinless chicken breasts

1 teaspoon hot pepper salsa

180 ml/6 fl oz chunky salsa

1. Grate the zest of the lemon and lime into a resealable bag. Squeeze the juice from both fruits into the bag, and throw out the pulp and the seeds.

2. Mix in everything else except the chicken and hot salsa.

3. Drop in the chicken, reseal the bag, and refrigerate for a few hours.

4. Grill the chicken, turning and basting with the marinade a few times, for 10 to 15 minutes or until the centre is no longer pink. Serve with salsa.

Makes 4 servings

Per serving: 184 calories/769 kJ; Protein 25 g; Carbs 11 g; Fat 5 g; Saturated fat 1 g; Sodium 740 mg; Fibre 2 g

Chilli-Peppered Steak (number of Powerfoods: 4)

1 tablespoon olive oil

2 carrots, sliced

1 large head broccoli, chopped

2 green chillies, sliced

2 red chillies, sliced

340 g/12 oz lean sirloin steak, thinly sliced

4 tablespoons chilli and garlic sauce

300 g/10½ oz brown rice, cooked

1. Heat the oil in a nonstick frying pan over a high heat. Toss in the carrots and broccoli, and cook until tender.

2. Add the chillies and beef, and continue cooking until the meat is done.

3. Add the sauce, and serve over the rice.

Makes 4 servings

Per serving: 520 calories/2184 kJ; Protein 33 g; Carbs 65 g; Fat 14 g; Saturated fat 4 g; Sodium 232 mg; Fibre 5 g

Philadelphia Fryers (number of Powerfoods: 3)

1 medium onion, sliced

1 small red pepper, sliced

1 small green pepper, sliced

150 ml/5 fl oz medium or hot salsa

4 multigrain rolls

340 g/12 oz roast beef, thinly sliced

60 g/2 oz reduced-fat Cheddar cheese, grated

1. In a nonstick frying pan over a medium heat, cook the onion and peppers until tender. Add the salsa and heat until warm.

2. Construct sandwiches with the rolls, roast beef, onions, peppers and cheese, then warm them in the microwave for 1 to 2 minutes on high, until the cheese starts to melt.

Makes 4 sandwiches

Per serving: 379 calories/1584 kJ; Protein 35 g; Carbs 35 g; Fat 12 g; Saturated fat 5 g; Sodium 442 mg; Fibre 5 g

Chilli Con Turkey (number of Powerfoods: 4)

455 g/1 lb minced turkey

1 can (400 g/14 oz) chopped tomatoes

1 can (400 g/14 oz) black beans, rinsed and drained

1 can (400 g/14 oz) sweetcorn, drained

45 g/1½ oz dried chilli mix

Dash of Tabasco

1 tablespoon ground flaxseed

4 tablespoons water

115 g/4 oz brown rice, cooked

1. In a large nonstick frying pan over a medium-high heat, brown the turkey.

2. Add everything else but the rice, and cook over a low heat for 10 minutes. Serve over the rice.

Makes 4 servings

Per serving: 480 calories/2006 kJ; Protein 41 g; Carbs 69 g; Fat 6 g; Saturated fat 1 g; Sodium 478 mg; Fibre 6 g

Chicken à la King Kong (number of Powerfoods: 3)

2 tablespoons olive oil

½ onion, finely chopped

1 teaspoon flour

2 tablespoons water

455 g/1 lb chicken breast fillets

4 teaspoons chilli powder

240 ml/8 fl oz pasta sauce

250 g/9 oz wholewheat spaghetti, cooked

1. Heat the oil in a nonstick frying pan over a medium-high heat. Add the onion and cook for 1 minute, until browned. In a small bowl, mix the flour and water.

2. Add the chicken, chilli powder, sauce and flour mixture to the frying pan. Stir. Simmer uncovered for 10 minutes. Serve over the spaghetti.

Makes 4 servings

Per serving: 286 calories/1195 kJ; Protein 30 g; Carbs 22 g; Fat 11 g; Saturated fat 2 g; Sodium 208 mg; Fibre 3.5 g

When You're Out

AT THE	EAT THIS	NOT THAT
Football game	Hot dog in a roll with ketchup: 450 cal., 18 g fat, 13 g protein	Cheeseburger with fries: 1,000 cal., 60 g fat, 30 g protein
Steakhouse	170-g/6-oz grilled rump steak, baked potato, ear of sweetcorn with pat of butter: 550 cal., 20 g fat, 55 g protein	6-oz rib eye steak, large portion of fries, 1 serving cauliflower cheese: 1,000 cal., 50 g fat, 60 g protein
Indian restaurant	Tandoori mixed grill; chickpea and spinach curry: 800 cal., 15 g fat, 28 g protein	2 poppadums with dips; chicken tikka masala with rice: 1,200 cal., 70 g fat, 60 g protein

Salmon Rushdie (number of Powerfoods: 5)

2 tablespoons olive oil

1 tablespoon lemon juice

¼ teaspoon salt

¼ teaspoon ground black pepper

1 tablespoon ground flaxseed

1 clove garlic, finely chopped

4 170-g/6-oz salmon fillets

Green vegetable of choice

115 g/4 oz brown rice, cooked

1. In a baking dish, combine the oil, lemon juice, salt, pepper, flaxseed and garlic. Add the fish, coat well, cover, and refrigerate for 15 minutes.

2. Preheat your oven to 230°C/450°F, gas 8. Line a baking sheet with foil, and coat it with cooking spray. Remove the fish from the marinade, and place the fish skin side down on the baking sheet.

3. Bake for 9 to 12 minutes. Serve with a green vegetable and rice.

Makes 4 servings

Per serving: 504 calories/2106 kJ; Protein 36 g; Carbs 25 g; Fat 29 g; Saturated fat 5 g; Sodium 470 mg; Fibre 3 g

BBQ King (number of Powerfoods: 5)

145 g/5 oz smoked turkey sausage, diced

1 small onion, chopped

90 g/3 oz mushrooms, sliced

1 clove garlic, finely chopped

1 can (415 g/15 oz) baked beans

1 can (225 g/8 oz) haricot or cannellini beans, drained

1 can (400 g/14 oz) chopped tomatoes

20 g/¾ oz seasoned breadcrumbs

¾ tablespoon ground flaxseed

¾ tablespoon olive oil

1. Preheat your oven to 180°C/350°F, gas 4. Put the sausage in a 2-litre baking dish, and bake until browned (about 5 minutes). Drain the fat and set the dish aside.

2. In a nonstick frying pan over a medium-high heat, cook the onion, mushrooms and garlic for 5 to 7 minutes. Transfer to the baking dish, then add the beans and tomatoes, plus salt and pepper to taste.

3. Bake for 20 minutes or until the edges bubble.

4. In a small bowl, mix the breadcrumbs and flaxseed with the oil. Sprinkle over the sausage mixture, and grill 10 to 13 cm/4 to 5 in from the heat until the top is golden (about 3 minutes).

Makes 4 servings

Per serving: 243 calories/1015 kJ; Protein 20 g; Carbs 31 g; Fat 6 g; Saturated fat 1 g; Sodium 1329 mg; Fibre 8 g

Spaghettaboudit! (number of Powerfoods: 3)

340 g/12 oz extra-lean minced beef

1½ onions, chopped

1 green pepper, chopped

2 cloves garlic, finely chopped

100 g/3½ oz mushrooms, sliced

2 cans (400 g/14 oz) peeled tomatoes

600 ml/20 fl oz pasta sauce

2 tablespoons Italian seasoning

455 g/1 lb wholewheat spaghetti

1. In a large saucepan over a medium-high heat, cook the meat until browned. Drain the fat from the meat.

2. Add the onion, green pepper and garlic, and cook until tender. Pour in the mushrooms, tomatoes (with their juice), sauce and seasoning, and stir everything together. Simmer. In a separate pot, cook the spaghetti according to the packet instructions.

3. Serve 120ml/4 fl oz of sauce over 115 g/4 oz of spaghetti.

Makes 4 servings

Per serving: 366 calories/1529 kJ; Protein 30 g; Carbs 48 g; Fat 8 g; Saturated fat 2 g; Sodium 801 mg; Fibre 7 g

Tortilla de Godzilla (number of Powerfoods: 4)

225 g/8 oz extra-lean minced beef or minced turkey

115 g/4 oz onion, chopped

2 cloves garlic, finely chopped

90 g/3 oz canned kidney beans, rinsed and mashed

2 green chilli peppers, seeded and diced

2 teaspoons chilli powder

4 large wholemeal tortillas

1 head lettuce, shredded

200 g/7 oz chopped tomatoes

30 g/1 oz low-fat Cheddar cheese, grated

1. In a large nonstick frying pan over a medium-high heat, cook the beef, onion and garlic until the beef is browned. Drain the fat.

2. Stir in the beans, chilli pepper and chilli powder, and cook until hot. Remove from the heat.

3. Warm the tortillas in the microwave for 20 seconds, then fill each tortilla with a quarter of the mixture. Top with lettuce, tomatoes and cheese, and roll each tortilla tightly into a tube.

Makes 4 servings

Per serving: 234 calories/978 kJ; Protein 20 g; Carbs 20 g; Fat 9 g; Saturated fat 5 g; Sodium 272 mg; Fibre 3 g

Abs Diet Snacks

Most diet plans portray snacking as a failure. I want you to think of snacking as exactly the opposite – as a key to success! But the secret to effective snacking is doing so at the optimum time – about 2 hours before you're scheduled to eat your next meal. That'll be enough time to head off hunger pangs and keep you full enough to avoid a meltdown at mealtime. You have a lot of flexibility in what you use to snack. You could have a portion of a leftover from dinner, a sandwich, a smoothie or a combination of some of the Abs Diet Powerfoods. To make it easier, pick one food from column A and one from column B. That will ensure your satiety.

A		B	
PROTEIN	**DAIRY**	**FRUIT OR VEGETABLE**	**COMPLEX CARBOHYDRATE**
2 teaspoons peanut butter (no added sugar)	225 g/8 oz low-fat yogurt	30 g/1 oz raisins	1 or 2 slices wholemeal bread
30 g/1 oz almonds	240 ml/8 fl oz skimmed milk or chocolate milk	Raw vegetables (celery, baby carrots, broccoli), unlimited	1 bowl hot oat or high-fibre cereal
3 thin slices turkey breast	180 ml/6 fl oz low-fat ice cream	170 g/6 oz berries	
3 thin slices roast beef	1½ slices low-fat cheese	115 g/4 oz cantaloupe melon	
	1 string cheese stick	1 large orange	
		1 can (330 ml/ 11½ fl oz) V8 juice	

Chapter 10

FITTING THE ABS DIET INTO EVERYDAY LIFE

How This Simple Eating Plan Makes Your Life Simpler, Too

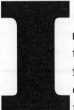N PREVIOUS CHAPTERS, I OUTLINED WHY the Abs Diet works – and will work for you, for life. I gave an overview of the science and fed you some nifty terms like *glycaemic index* and *basal metabolism*. And I listed a whole eating plan complete with meals, snacks and simple recipes.

But I also explained why most other diet plans are the nutritional equivalent of that tape recorder in *Mission: Impossible* – programmed to self-destruct in 5 seconds, or 5 weeks, or 5 years. Most diets just aren't designed to last over the long haul, or they're so complicated and restrictive that you'd have to quit your day job and disown half your friends in order to follow them to the letter. Many diets fail because they require us to work too hard and ignore the fact that we're already working too hard. What most of us feel, every day, is that our worlds are on the verge of spinning out of control. And what we want is to take back control: to take control of our lives, our careers, our relationships, our bodies, our diets, ourselves.

That's why I want to take a break at this point and demonstrate for you how easily the Abs Diet fits into a busy lifestyle and how adopting its simple eating strategies can take a lot of the work, stress and hassle out of everyday life. To do that, I've decided to give you a quick profile of a day in the life of a typical hardworking guy. Let's call him Joe.

A Day in the Life of Joe

6.30 AM Joe wakes up, staggers out to the kitchen, and starts the coffeepot. While the coffee's brewing, he pulls a mug out of a cabinet and fills it with skimmed milk. He drinks the milk down until there's about 2 tablespoons left, then pours in the coffee.[1] Then he grabs the papers and flips through them quickly, stopping at the obituaries just in case he died the night before and nobody told him.

7 AM Joe turns on the morning talk shows, and while the goofy smiling weatherman tells him what's in store for the day, he takes some ice, some yogurt, a spoonful each of whey protein and ground flaxseed, plus some leftover fruit and maybe some lime juice or orange juice or whatever else happens to be lying around the kitchen, and throws the whole menagerie into a blender. He buzzes that into oblivion for 30 seconds, pours some into a glass, and pours

---

1. A blast of low-fat protein and calcium gives you an immediate metabolic boost and helps ensure you get your daily quota of calcium and vitamin D. The coffee cup ritual is just a good reminder to have that glass of low-fat milk every morning.

the rest of it into a small flask, which he will carry to his office.[2]

8 AM Having showered, shaved and dressed, Joe leaves his house and walks to work, which takes about 35 minutes. On the way, he stops at a grocery shop and grabs a little packet of almonds and an apple, which he sticks in his desk. He puts his Thermos of smoothie into the fridge in the office kitchen. Then he goes through his work – returns phone calls, answers e-mail and the like.

10 AM While he's *still* returning e-mail (ugh), he snacks on the almonds and fruit. That tides him over till lunchtime.[3]

Noon If Joe can, he skips out to the gym. (He avoids business lunches as much as possible; they suck time out of his day and suck control away from his diet.)

1 PM He'll usually grab a protein bar or protein shake at the gym.[4] Then he'll stroll over to the soup-and-sandwich joint, where he'll order a take-out spinach salad that's loaded with beans, sweetcorn, broccoli, red peppers and tandoori chicken and topped with a half-ladle of balsamic vinegar.[5]

---

2. More protein, more calcium, plus fibre, vitamins and minerals. By making a little extra and taking it to work, Joe manages to prepare two food opportunities in about 30 seconds. (*Note* A little portable jug cooler keeps the smoothie's consistency – even if you put the blender glass in the fridge, the smoothie tends to separate after a few hours and become chalky.)

3. More fibre and more vitamins, minerals and protein. I can't stress enough the importance of stashing food in your office. Trail mix, dehydrated high-fibre soups and cereals and fruit are staples of a workday diet. Once you stock your office with healthy snacks, you have seized control of your workday. When a meeting runs over and you can't get out for lunch, you've got healthy food on hand. Again, the more control you have over your food, the more you have over your body, and the more you have over your life.

4. More and more research indicates the importance of eating immediately after your workout, when your body is searching around for an energy source. If you eat immediately, your body uses the food to rebuild muscle; if you stay hungry, your body breaks down muscle for energy, and that's not good. I don't even like to wait the 10 minutes it takes between the gym and the takeaway; I eat immediately after my workout (though not in the locker room, which is just too gross).

5. More fibre, more protein, more vitamins and minerals. We're beginning to detect a pattern, Captain.

3 PM Joe's hungry (again). Fortunately, he's got a delicious smoothie hidden away in the office fridge. While others might be hitting their 3 PM slump, he's hitting the smoothie for a quick burst of energy.[6]

7.30 PM For the past 5 hours, Joe's been grinding away at work, so naturally he's ready for . . . more work. Joe has a business dinner almost every night. Dinner is his least disciplined part of the day, but the Abs Diet is pretty forgiving: his typical dinner starts with a salad, then moves onto a rump steak with a side dish of broccoli or green beans.[7] On top of that, he'll have a couple

---

6. Yes, yes, we know . . . more protein, more calcium, more fibre. Does this guy ever stop?

7. Order the steak; skip the mashed potatoes. A lot of us like to eat a lot at dinner, so at this meal, you simply keep carbs restricted as much as you can. That way, you can eat as much as you want.

ABS DIET SUCCESS STORY

'I SOLVED MY BACK PAIN – AND REGAINED MY LIFE!'

Name: Steve Toomey

Age: 39

Height: 1.91 m/6'3"

Starting weight: 97.5 kg/15 st 5 lb

Six weeks later: 88.5 kg/13 st 13 lb

When Steve Toomey rolled around in bed, he'd feel his back tense up at the slightest movement. It wasn't excruciating pain, but it was annoying – and it was interfering with his life.

'It really hampered my ability to play with my kids,' he says. 'I have one who's 6, one who's 5, one who's 3, and one on the way, and all they want to do is wrestle and roll around on the floor. All they were saying was, "Daddy, when is your back going to get better so we can wrestle?"'

of glasses of red wine and maybe dessert – although he usually shares it.[8]

11 PM At home, Joe will often start grubbing around his refrigerator for something more to nosh on. He usually keeps a couple of different types of cold cuts in there – turkey, Gruyère, and a glass of skimmed milk will often complete his night.[9]

8. Yes, it's OK to have dessert. Remember that high-fat, high-sugar foods are for indulging, not for mindless snacking. I'd rather you order the crème brûlée at a restaurant and really love it than mindlessly down half a bag of crisps while watching TV – hundreds of fatty, salty calories that you won't remember eating 10 minutes later. Share the dessert with someone so that you get all the pleasure and half the guilt. (Note: your pleasure-to-guilt ratio may vary depending on who you're sharing that dessert with.)

9. More calcium and more protein, including tryptophan, which is found in turkey and dairy products and helps induce sleep.

A doctor told him he needed to stretch his back. When he went back and said that stretching wasn't helping, the doctor told him to give it one more chance and then they'd take an MRI. But that's when he started the Abs Diet.

'Once I incorporated the abs routine, the pain was gone,' Toomey says. 'Now I'm religious about the plan.'

Since he started the programme, he's lost 6 cm/2½ inches from his waist, and he no longer has pain at night or fear that he's going to pull something when he's playing with the kids.

And in a house full of kids, where pizza and hot dogs are always on hand, Toomey has also appreciated the change in diet.

'The diet isn't nearly as restrictive as some of the diets I've tried, particularly the [ones with] super-low carbohydrates,' he says. 'On them, I used to crave slices of bread. Here, I can eat some carbs. I'm never starving or super hungry.' But the biggest reward might be that weekly cheat meal. 'My wife makes these Vietnamese egg rolls that are deep-fried, which I love. So I've been able to eat those on Sundays and not feel guilty,' Toomey says. 'I think that's really key – to be able to cheat once a week and know you're not going to ruin anything.'

How Stress Makes You Fat

One of the great side benefits of the Abs Diet is that it helps you take control of your life, which means taking control of your stress level. I can't emphasize strongly enough how important stress management is for your weight, for your health and for the quality of life you'll lead.

That's because our bodies simply aren't designed to handle the stress of modern life. See, when stress hits, one of the first things your body does is jack up its production of adrenalin. Adrenalin causes fat cells all over your body to squirt their stores of fatty acids into your bloodstream to be used as energy. This was great back when stress meant a charging sabre-toothed tiger or an attacking horde of barbarians and your fight-or-flight mechanism switched on. But it's not so great in today's society, where the only tigers and barbarians you have to handle are the ones who sign your pay-cheque. You don't flee or fight; you just knuckle down to get that report finished and munch your way through a midnight deadline. Meanwhile, your adrenal glands are producing yet another hormone to handle all that freshly released fat. It's called cortisol, but I want you to call it by its nickname: the tummy-fat hormone.

In one Yale study, researchers asked 42 overweight people to perform an hour of stressful tasks – maths problems, puzzles and speech making. All the while, their cortisol levels were measured. The subjects who carried their extra weight in their stomachs were discovered to be secreting more cortisol while under pressure. The theory runs like this: stress hits, adrenalin mobilizes fat from all over the body, and cortisol takes the unused portion and stashes it with extreme prejudice towards the abdominal region. In a study of 438 male firefighters, the ones who said they worried about their financial security gained 5 kg/11.2 pounds over 7 years, compared with an average of 3.3 kg/7.4 lb gained by non-worriers. The key to managing your midsection, then, is managing your stress. Here are a few proven ways to keep your head – and your abs – when all around you are losing theirs.

Skip late-night TV. A University of Chicago study published in the journal *Sleep* showed that men who slept only 4 hours a night had cortisol levels 37 per cent higher than men who got a full 8 hours of shut-eye; the men who stayed awake the whole night had levels 45 per cent higher. Sleep specialists suggest that you strive for 8 hours per night.

Stop tossing and turning. How well you sleep matters, too. Another University of Chicago study showed that men who got plenty of deep sleep – the quality stuff without all the dreaming and rapid eye movement – secreted almost 65 per cent more human growth hormone (HGH) than men who were short on good slumber. You want more HGH to help prevent the loss of muscle mass caused by cortisol.

Remember C, as in 'crisis'. If you're in a stressful time of life – wondering why the jury has been out so long, perhaps – load up on vitamin C. For managing stress, you probably maximize the benefit with a daily intake of 1,000 milligrams, divided into small doses throughout the day.

Don't have that last drink. Booze dehydrates you. Your body

SNEAKY WAYS TO KEEP RESTAURANTS FROM SABOTAGING YOUR DIET

Many chefs pour at least 30 g/1 oz of butter (200 calories and 23 grams of fat) onto a steak just so the meat will look juicier. Ask in advance, and tell the cook to lay off.

Those harmless-looking shredded carrots that dress up your beef are probably deep-fried; 60 g/2 oz is 137 calories (four times that of raw carrots) and 12 grams of fat. Skip 'em.

If you go to a restaurant that serves salads tossed with dressing, it's usually a much lighter coating than what most people end up dumping on themselves, even if you order it on the side.

thinks there's a water shortage emergency, which bumps up your cortisol. How much alcohol is too much? Most of the smart money says three drinks a day. Same dehydration idea applies to caffeine. For cortisol control, stick to 200 milligrams per day, about what you get in two cups of coffee.

Take the wheel. A sense of control over some of the stressors in your life helps. 'If you blast a volunteer randomly with a noise, his stress hormones rise,' says Dr Robert Sapolsky, professor of biological and neurological sciences at Stanford University. 'But if you give him a button and tell him that pressing it will decrease the likelihood of the noise, there's a smaller stress response to the same sound.' Getting organized, even in small ways, may help you feel more like the captain of your ship.

Make a plan. 'People manage stress more effectively if they can believe that things are improving,' says Sapolsky. So make sure you always have something you're looking forward to. Hope makes stress manageable.

Get spiritual. Remember the simple wisdom of Simone Weil: Any undivided attention is prayer. If we can stop the tumble in our heads and every day briefly commit our complete attention to something – a 3-m/10-foot putt, completing a crossword or a 10-year-old child – we may acquire the serenity many find in formal faith.

Chapter II

TURBOCHARGING THE ABS DIET

How Exercise Can Strip Away Fat and Add Muscle

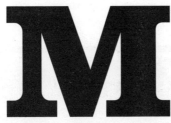**AYBE THE LAST FEW** months, years, or decades of your life have been one big snowstorm – a snowstorm of office parties and happy hours, of vending machine dinners, of midnight pizza deliveries. When you're a kid, those storms can be fun, but as you get older, they're more of a mess than anything else. They dump unwelcome amounts of fat onto your once-svelte gut, leaving your abs buried deep under everything. No sun's going to melt your fat after a couple of days, and no snowblower's going to suck it up and shoot it over to the neighbour's lawn. (But how cool would that be?)

If you want to see the pavement, you have to shovel the snow. If you want to find your abs, you have to burn the fat.

Eating right is critical and, yes, by following the nutrition principles of the Abs Diet and centring your meals around the Abs Diet Powerfoods, you'll lose fat pretty effortlessly. But to maximize your weight loss and turn your fat into muscle, this book includes something other diet books ignore: a quick-and-easy exercise plan. Exercise will not only make you healthier; it'll make you lose weight faster. It'll make you stronger. Most important, it'll make your body turn fat into muscle – by converting energy that's stored in fat into energy that feeds muscle.

The Abs Diet Workout Principles

HAVING WORKED AT *Men's Health* for more than 15 years, I know all the latest trends in exercise, but I also scour the latest and most credible scientific research measuring the effectiveness of

ABS DIET SUCCESS STORY

'I REGAINED MY SELF-ESTEEM!'

Name: Brian Archiquette
Age: 35
Height: 1.91 m/ 6' 3"
Starting weight: 124.7 kg/ 19 st 9 lb
Six weeks later: 113.4kg/ 17 st 12 lb

After reaching his all-time high of 156.5 kg/ 24 st 9 lb, Brian Archiquette signed up for the gym. He had steadily gained 59 kg/ 9 st 4 lb after getting married 9 years ago, and he had finally had it. He was tired of being fat. He felt miserable and depressed. 'I felt like I was standing on the sidelines of life,' he says.

Add in the fact that his father died of congestive heart failure and that he was headed in the same direction, and Archiquette knew he had to make a change – and he'd have to do it now. He followed workouts in *Men's Health* magazine and various workout plans. With that knowledge, I've constructed the exercise portion of the plan to help you burn fat at the highest levels possible in the least amount of time. I know you don't have time to spend hours a day exercising, so I want you to get the most out of every workout. And I know that flexibility and convenience are the keys to formulating a plan you can stick to, so I've created a workout you can do in your local gym – or in your living room. This plan allows you to keep your workouts short and focused, while still keeping you on target for your ultimate goal. It's the best workout possible for finding your abs. These are the workout principles.

Focus on your diet first. The first 2 weeks of exercise are optional. If you already exercise regularly, you can jump right into the Abs Diet Workout, and you should, because you'll burn even more fat than with the Abs Diet alone. But if you're a beginner or you haven't exercised in a long time, take the first 2 weeks to adjust to your new eating plan before starting the workout. If

gradually dropped to 124.7 kg/ 19 st 9 lb. When he went on the Abs Diet, he supercharged the weight loss and dropped an additional 11.3 kg/ 25 lb in 6 weeks.

'It was planning the meals and the timing of the meals. I was trying to balance the meals throughout the day, plus add the exercise,' says Archiquette, whose weakness is pizza. 'In the past, what would happen is that I wouldn't eat, and then I'd overeat because I got so hungry.'

While he's on his way to reaching his goal of weighing 97.5 kg/ 15 st 5 lb on his 1.91-m/ 6ft 3-in frame, he's already made tremendous gains. He's dropped from a 122-cm/ 48-in waist to a 102-cm/ 40-in waist. And now when he walks through a shopping centre, he doesn't have to find a place to sit down every couple of minutes. The biggest gain, he says, has been in his self-esteem.

'I definitely have more energy and a more positive outlook on life,' he says. 'I'm more confident – even when I'm standing in front of people at work. I was always self-conscious, thinking that they're looking at my stomach sticking out or that my shirt is too tight. Now I feel better about myself.'

you're champing at the bit to begin maximizing your weight loss, start getting in the exercise habit by walking briskly for up to 30 minutes a day.

Focus on muscles. I used to work with a guy who was about 13.6 kg/ 30 lb overweight. He decided he'd enter a race as motivation to help him lose weight. He ran 6 days a week and followed his running programme religiously, but he didn't lose anything. Sure, he was able to run further than he ever had, but his body stayed the same. Why? First, because he still based his diet around pizza, pasta and burgers, and secondly, because steady-state cardiovascular exercise doesn't burn fat the way strength training does. (Incidentally, when the same guy went on the Abs Diet and started a weightlifting programme, he lost nearly 9 kg/ 20 lb in less than 2 months.)

Your muscles are hungry little suckers, and in order to keep themselves well nourished, they want to churn and burn those cal-

ABSFACTS

Stay slow and steady

Here's a trick: slowly say the phrase 'slow and controlled' to yourself as you curl your body upwards during an abdominal crunch. It should take at least as much time to reach the top of the movement as it does to say this mantra (same goes for the way down).

Stretch it out

If your hamstrings are tight, you may develop a habit of leaning backwards to relieve the pressure. This posture tends to thrust your gut forwards, making your paunch look even paunchier. Stretching your hamstrings a few times a week should help. If you're already stretched – for time, that is – the fastest way to loosen up your back and hamstrings and tighten your abdomen is by doing what's called the Figure-4 Stretch. Here's how to do it: sit on the floor with your right leg straight in front of you, toes pointing up. Bend your left knee to place your left heel against the inside of your right thigh, near your groin; keep your left knee almost touching the floor. Now reach out slowly with your right arm and touch your right toe. If you can't do it, try grabbing your ankle. Hold the position for 30 seconds, return to the starting position, and then stretch again for another 30 seconds. Switch legs, and stretch your left side twice also.

ories you're ingesting. So the more muscle you have, the more calories you burn – in the gym, on the job, even in bed. This programme focuses on working your large muscle groups – your legs, chest, back and shoulders – because that's where you can build the most muscle in the least amount of time. Plus, when you work your larger muscles, you fire up your metabolism by creating a longer calorie afterburn – one that can last right up to your very next workout!

Think about the small fraction of time you spend exercising. Even if you work out four or five times a day for an hour at a time, that's nothing compared to the amount of time you're not exercising every day. So in order to gain the most metabolic benefit, you want to maximize the calories you're burning when you're not working out.

Focus on spending less time in the gym. The Abs Diet Workout employs two simple concepts to maximize muscle growth and fat-burning and minimize the time you spend exercising.

Kick the butts

Research shows that smokers have a greater abdomen-to-hip ratio than former smokers or people who never smoked. That means smokers are more likely to put on weight around their midsections. It's yet another reason to put down those cancer sticks for good.

Think small

Sure, excess calories lead to excess weight. But how and when you eat are just as important as what. Eating large meals, for example, can actually stretch your abdominal muscles outwards. Stuff yourself on a regular basis, and your abs will become so stretched that they'll lose their ability to rein in your gut. That's another reason why multiple small meals are better than a few large ones.

Get some flex time

When you're sitting in your car or at your desk, tense your middle as you would at the start of the crunch. Sit up straight and pull your abs in for 60 seconds at a time, at least once an hour. Anytime you feel them going slack throughout your day, tighten them up again.

Circuit training. This term refers to the practice of performing different exercises one right after another. For example, we'll have you do a set of leg exercises followed immediately by a set of an upper-body exercise, until you do 8 to 10 different exercises in a row. There are two reasons circuit training works. First, by keeping you moving and cutting down the rest periods between exercises, circuit training keeps your heart rate elevated throughout your training session, maximizing your fat burn while providing tremendous cardiovascular fitness benefits. Secondly, circuit training keeps your workout short – you won't waste time resting between sets of an exercise, which means you can get on with the rest of your busy life.

Compound exercises. Another key part of the strength-training programme is compound exercises, that is, exercises that call into play multiple muscle groups rather than just focusing on

---

ABSFACTS

Stand tall

When you're walking, stand tall and picture a cape flowing off your shoulders, Superman-style, to ensure your best posture. A taller posture will give you the appearance of being slimmer, while also training your abs to stay taut and firm. Another good trick is to think of your back as a wall and your gut as a piece of furniture pushed up against the wall to keep it from buckling.

Watch your back

Contrary to popular belief, your abs aren't found just around your navel. They're an intricate system of muscles, connecting to your rib cage, your hips, and even your backbone. To have strong abs, you need not only stomach exercises but also lower-back strength and exercises for your obliques (the abdominal muscles that run down the sides of your torso).

Tune in to muscle

Maybe you've heard of 'muscle memory': the way your body learns to do a physical activity (like riding a bike) and never forgets. Well, your abs have a

one. For example, with the Abs Diet Workout, we don't want you to exercise your chest, and then your shoulders, and then your triceps, and then your forearms. We want you to hit many different muscles at the same time and then get out of the gym. One study showed that you can put on 2.76 kb/ 6 lb of muscle and lose 6.8 kg/ 15 lb of fat in 6 weeks by following an exercise programme that employs the compound exercises found in the Abs Diet Workout. What's even better is that those subjects followed an exercise plan for only 20 minutes three times a week. Not only do compound exercises make your workout more fun and more challenging, they will also increase the demands on your muscles – even though you're not actually doing more work. (For instance, the squat hits a whopping 256 muscles with just one movement!) Greater muscle demand triggers your body to produce more human growth hormone – a potent fat burner.

memory, too. If you consciously keep your abs firm throughout the day, they'll tend to stay firm even when you're relaxed.

Put exercise first

Research suggests that the best way to eat less at a meal is to work out right before it. This works in several ways: firstl you're less hungry when your metabolism is revving, such as right after a workout. Secondly, you're thirstier, so you drink more water, which uses up space in your stomach and relieves hunger. Thirdly, with your metabolism revved, the calories you do eat get burned for energy pronto – not stored as fat.

Avoid the four-letter word

When you lose weight on a 'diet', muscle is the first thing to go. It's more expensive for your body to retain than fat is, so when you run low on calories, your body dumps muscle mass and turns it into energy. When you go off the diet, you begin to gain back the weight – but because you now have less calorie-burning muscle, the weight you gain is fat. By dieting, you've effectively turned muscle into fat.

By working more muscle, your body uses more energy to repair and upgrade it the day after your workout. A 2008 US study showed that people burned more calories the day after they did lower-body resistance training than the day after they worked their upper bodies, simply because the leg muscles generally have more mass than the muscles in the chest and arms.

If the only weight you've ever picked up is around your gut and not in the gym, don't worry that you're not familiar with working with weights. You can start by lifting any amount of weight that you're comfortable with – whether it's a pair of light dumbbells or a couple of cans of beans. Even if you start small, you'll grow stronger, start to build muscle, and keep your metabolism revved. As you progress, you'll build and burn more.

Focus on intensity. Go back to the guy I worked with. He ran 6 days a week, but he ran as slow as the ketchup at the bottom of the bottle. His intensity never elevated, and because of that, he never burned that much fat. Time and time again, research has shown that higher-intensity workouts promote weight loss better than steady-state activities. In a Canadian study from Laval University, researchers measured differences in fat loss between two groups of exercisers following two different workout programmes. The first group rode stationary bikes four or five times a week and burned 300 to 400 calories per 30- to 45-minute session. The second group did the same, but only one or two times a week, and they filled the rest of their sessions with short intervals of high-intensity cycling. They hopped on their stationary bikes and pedalled as quickly as they could for 30 to 90 seconds, rested, and then repeated the process several times per exercise session. As a result, they burned 225 to 250 calories while cycling, but they had burned more fat at the end of the study than the workers in the first group. In fact, even though they exercised less, their fat loss was nine times greater. Researchers said that the majority of the fat burning took place after the workout.

The Abs Diet Workout recommends that you add one simple interval workout per week to complement your strength training. These are workouts of traditional cardiovascular exercise (running, swimming, biking) in which you alternate between periods of high intensity and periods of rest. (I'll explain more about how to create an effective interval workout in the next chapter.)

If You Don't Already Exercise

THE BEST PART about the 6-week Abs Diet Workout is that, for the first 2 weeks at least, you don't actually have to exercise. If you're not doing anything right now, it's not critical that you start immediately. Instead, I want you to concentrate on acclimatizing your body and your schedule to the Abs Diet.

On the other hand, why wait to fire up your fat-burning mechanisms? If you want to start a light strength-training programme, do this workout three times a week: alternate between three sets of Press-ups and three sets of Squats with no weights. Both exercises use your body weight as resistance and will get your body accustomed to a strength-training programme. Do 8 to 10 repetitions of Press-ups, followed by 15 to 20 repetitions of Squats. When that becomes too easy, increase the repetitions of Press-ups, and use some form of weight – light dumbbells are best – while doing Squats. This light workout, especially in combination with 30 minutes of brisk walking, will really fire up your fat burners.

If You're Already in the Exercise Habit

MAYBE YOU LIFT weights once or twice a week. Maybe you jog a few miles every morning. Maybe you're a pretty good swimmer. I dunno. What I do know is that no matter what your workout is now, you're probably going to build more muscle, and burn more fat, if you switch to the Abs Diet Workout.

Even if your current exercise programme has been working well for you, experts agree that mixing up your workout every month or so is the best way to maximize your results. That's because gains in strength and overall fitness come from challenging your body to perform in ways it's not used to. Performing the same workout over and over again doesn't train your body to reach its potential; it just trains your body to be really, really good at performing that one workout. So I want you to consider switching your current workout over to the Abs Diet Workout, at least for a few weeks. I guarantee the results you'll see will be astounding.

Suggested Weekly Workout Schedule

YOU CAN MIX and match the different workouts to meet your lifestyle needs. When you construct your schedule, make sure to:

▶ Leave at least 48 hours between weight workouts of the same body parts. Your muscles need time to recover and repair themselves after a workout.

▶ Take 1 day each week to rest with no formal exercise.

▶ Warm up for 5 minutes before starting to exercise, through gentle jogging, riding on a stationary bike, skipping or doing slow jumping jacks.

The three components of your weekly schedule include:

1. Strength training: Three times a week. These are total-body workouts with one workout that puts extra emphasis on your legs.

2. Additional cardiovascular work: Optional, on non-strength-training days. Try cycling, running, swimming and using cardio machines. An interval workout is recommended for 1 day a week, and light cardiovascular exercise like walking is recommended for 2 of your 3 off days.

3. Abs exercises: Twice a week. Do them before strength training or interval workouts (see chapter 13).

Chapter 12

THE ABS DIET WORKOUT

The Easiest, Most Effective Workout Plan Ever

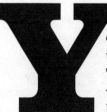**OU SEE EVERY KIND OF PERSON IN** the gym. The guy with no fat. The guy with no neck. The guy with lots of fat. The guy with lots of necks. And it seems they all get there a different way. I know that guys have as many different workout philosophies as they have pirated MP3 files, but the one guy I really know I can help is the overweight man who's working his forearm muscles by doing wrist curls in the corner. He's like a guy who has totalled his car but wants to get the radio fixed first. There's no point working on the fine points until you've taken care of the bigger issues.

That's why I've built a total-body strength training workout: to increase your lean muscle mass as efficiently as possible. It's simple: to show off your abs, you have to burn fat. To burn fat, you have to build muscle. Remember that adding just ½ kg/ 1 lb of muscle will force your body to burn up to an additional 50 calories a day, every day.

This workout emphasizes the larger muscle groups of your body – chest, back and legs. In one workout during the week, you'll give extra attention to your legs. I know what you're thinking: my abs are up here. Why do I care about working what's down there? Because most of your body's muscle is found below your tummy button. Your lower body is where you'll build the most muscle in the least amount of time; working this giant muscle mass triggers the release of large amounts of growth hormone, which in turn stimulates muscle growth throughout your body, kicks your fat burners into overdrive, and gives you that washboard stomach you want – in no time flat. Indeed, leg exercises are the key to total-body strength: in one Norwegian study, men who focused on lower-body work gained more upper-body strength than did those who emphasized upper-body exercises in their workouts. That doesn't mean you'll ignore your upper body entirely, though. With the upper-body workout, you'll also work your largest muscles – your chest, back and shoulders – to burn more fat. If you follow this programme, you'll still notice more growth and definition in your whole body – even your forearms, even your shoulders and, yes, even your abs – and you'll begin to reshape your body.

Here, you're going to do circuit training to optimize your muscle-building potential. That is, you'll perform one set of an exercise and then move immediately to the next exercise, with just 30 seconds of rest. Follow the order of the exercises I've listed on the following pages; that will allow you to work different body parts from set to set. (A complete set of exercise descriptions and instructional photos begins on page 192.) By alternating between body parts, you'll keep your body in constant work mode and be able to perform the movements back-to-back without rest. Here's why circuit training works so well: you'll save time because you'll cut the amount of rest you need when you alternate muscle groups. More importantly, you'll keep your heart rate elevated throughout the workout, so you'll burn even more fat while you're exercising – whether it's in the gym or in your own living room.

In the first 2 weeks of the programme, do the circuit twice. Move from exercise to exercise with no more than 30 seconds of rest in between. When you complete one circuit, rest for 1 to 2 minutes, then complete the second circuit. After the first 2 weeks, when you've become comfortable doing two complete circuits in a workout, increase your workload to three circuits per workout. In every exercise, use a weight that you can handle comfortably for the number of repetitions noted. When that becomes too easy, increase the weight on each set by 10 per cent or less. Here's a sample schedule of how you might arrange your workouts.

MONDAY
Total-Body Strength Training Workout with Ab Emphasis
Complete one set of each ab exercise*,
then complete the rest of the circuit twice.

EXERCISE	REPETITIONS	REST	SETS
Traditional Crunch* (page 221)	12–15	none	1
Bent-Leg Knee Raise* (page 231)	12–15	none	1
Oblique V-Up* (page 241)	10 each side	none	1
Bridge* (page 247)	1 or 2	none	1
Back Extension* (page 255)	12–15	none	1
Squat	10–12	30 seconds	2
Bench Press	10	30 seconds	2
Pulldown	10	30 seconds	2
Military Press	10	30 seconds	2
Upright Row	10	30 seconds	2
Triceps Pushdown	10–12	30 seconds	2
Leg Extension	10–12	30 seconds	2
Biceps Curl	10	30 seconds	2
Leg Curl	10–12	30 seconds	2

TUESDAY (Optional)
**Light Cardiovascular Exercise Such as Walking
(Try for 30 Minutes at a Brisk Pace)**

WEDNESDAY
Total-Body Strength Training Workout with Ab Emphasis
Complete one set of each ab exercise* once,
then complete rest of circuit twice.

EXERCISE	REPETITIONS	REST	SETS
Standing Crunch* (page 222)	12–15	none	1
Pulse Up* (page 232)	12	none	1
Saxon Side Bend* (page 242)	6–10 each side	none	1
Side Bridge* (page 248)	1 or 2 each side	none	1
Back Extension* (page 255)	12–15	none	1
Squat	10–12	30 seconds	2
Bench Press	10	30 seconds	2
Pulldown	10	30 seconds	2
Military Press	10	30 seconds	2
Upright Row	10	30 seconds	2
Triceps Pushdown	10–12	30 seconds	2
Leg Extension	10–12	30 seconds	2
Biceps Curl	10	30 seconds	2
Leg Curl	10–12	30 seconds	2

THURSDAY (Optional)
**Light Cardiovascular Exercise Such as Walking
(Try for 30–45 Minutes at a Brisk Pace)**

FRIDAY
Total-Body Strength Training Workout, with Leg Emphasis
Repeat entire circuit twice.

EXERCISE	REPETITIONS	REST	SETS
Squat	10–12	30 seconds	2
Bench Press	10	30 seconds	2
Pulldown	10	30 seconds	2
Travelling Lunge	10–12 each leg	30 seconds	2
Military Press	10	30 seconds	2
Upright Row	10	30 seconds	2
Step-Up	10–12 each leg	30 seconds	2
Triceps Pushdown	10–12	30 seconds	2
Leg Extension	10–12	30 seconds	2
Biceps Curl	10	30 seconds	2
Leg Curl	10–12	30 seconds	2

SATURDAY (Optional)
Abs Workout Plus Interval Workout
Complete one set of each ab exercise, then choose
one interval workout from the selection on pages 214 and 215.

EXERCISE	REPETITIONS	REST	SETS
Traditional Crunch (page 221)	12–15	None	1
Bent-Leg Knee Raise (page 231	12	None	1
Oblique V-Up (page 241)	6–10 each side	None	1
Bridge (page 247)	1–2	None	1
Back Extension (page 255)	12–15	None	1

SUNDAY Off

BURN FAT FASTER WITH EXERCISE MACHINES

While I'm a big believer in building muscle to burn fat, working out on cardio machines can help you lose lard, too – but only if you use them correctly. Most of the time, however, people expend too much time and silly-looking movement for too small a payoff.

The huge benefit to machines is that they allow you to work very hard in a very short time period. They can make a lunchtime workout an exercise in efficiency or make a pre-work morning session not only possible but effective as well. Fix the common exercise machine mistakes below, and you'll burn more fat than the sweat-spraying cardio crazies with the blurry legs and burning lungs . . . and still have time for a smoothie afterwards.

1. TREADMILL.
• Your Form
The mistake: Too much bouncing up and down. Your head should remain relatively level while running otherwise you'll tire out your joints – and yourself – too soon.
The fix: Improve flexibility to smooth out your stride. Try leg swings – hold the handlebar, stand on one leg, and swing the other back and forth, keeping your upper body still. This will loosen and warm you up, making your legs more pliable.
• Your Workout
The mistake: Too many long, steady, flat runs.
The fix: Run shorter and harder, mixing speeds and inclines to create intervals. You'll fatigue your muscles and your energy source more quickly, leading to more efficient fat burning throughout the day. Start with a 2 per cent incline, and over several sessions work up to 10 per cent. (Just walk at this point.) The more intense the workout, the shorter it can be.

2. STATIONARY BIKE
• Your Form
The mistake: The seat is too low or too high. A very low seat fatigues the legs a lot more and adds stress on the knees. Set it too high and your hips rock from side to side, which is uncomfortable and inefficient, and makes you look funny.
The fix: Adjust the seat, people! Sit on the seat and place your heel in the middle of the pedal, where the ball of your foot would normally go. You want your leg fully extended, straight down, at the lowest point of the pedal rotation. By moving your foot to the correct position on the pedal, you'll have the right amount of bend.
• Your Workout
The mistake: Cruising instead of charging.
The fix: Vary the intensity, with 2 to 3 minutes of high-cadence pedalling and a 3-minute recovery, then repeat for 15 minutes. Stand occasionally, which

will add another dimension to your workout. Standing requires more muscle not only to push the pedals, but also to support and balance your body.

3. ROWING MACHINE

• Your Form

The mistake: Your hands bump your knees, and throws off your cadence.

The fix: Take a tip from rowing crews to create a fluid motion: Think of the stroke as a dance, counting 1-2-3 and 3-2-1. On 1, push with your legs; on 2, 'swing up' your body by leaning back; on 3, draw your arms to the bottom of your rib cage, spinning the flywheel. Then reverse it: 3, extend your arms; 2, swing your body forward from the hips; 1, bring your legs up after the handle passes your knees.

• Your Workout

The mistake: A long, steady slog, which leads to inefficient exercise.

The fix: With medium resistance, do four to six 10-minute sets of rowing with 2 to 3 minutes of rest in between. This will allow your heart rate to come down a bit so you regroup and start fresh with intense effort.

4. ELLIPTICAL TRAINER

* Your Form

The mistake: Too little resistance. It's common for people to allow momentum to work for them instead of propelling the step with their leg muscles.

The fix: Set the resistance correctly. Gliding isn't good. You want to be able to feel that you are pushing the ramp down when you make a revolution rather than flipping around freely.

As your balance improves, keep your hands at your sides; you'll recruit core muscles to keep yourself stable.

• Your Workout

The mistake: Falling into boring ruts.

The fix: Do intervals. It will force you to reach a higher intensity of training for a sustained period of time. Try 90-second blasts every few minutes, with recoveries twice as long. Reduce recovery time as your fitness level increases.

5. STAIRCLIMBER

• Your Form

The mistake: Holding yourself up with your arms. A lot of people put their hands on the railing and lock their elbows with arms straight down. That's like using crutches.

The fix: Rest your hands lightly on the bars only for balance. Keep your body upright, with just a slight lean forward as if you are leaning to walk up a flight of stairs.

• Your Workout

The mistake: Too little resistance.

The fix: Go slower, with challenging resistance. You'll give yourself a tougher workout, increase your heart rate and maintain your time in the training zone longer. Result: You'll burn more fat.

BASIC EXERCISES

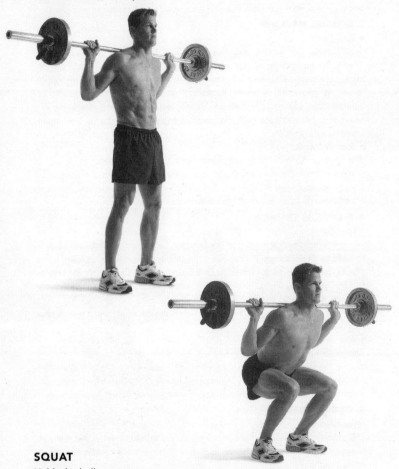

SQUAT

Hold a barbell
with an overhand grip so that it rests comfortably on your upper back. Set
your feet shoulder-width apart, and keep your knees slightly bent, back
straight, and eyes focused straight ahead. Slowly lower your body as if you
were sitting back into a chair, keeping your back in its natural
alignment and your lower legs nearly perpendicular to the floor. When your
thighs are parallel to the floor, pause, then return to the starting position.

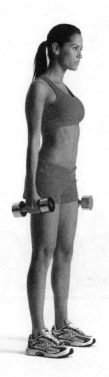

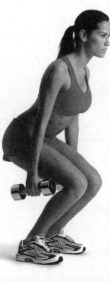

HOME VARIATION: *Same, but with one dumbbell in each hand, your palms facing your outer thighs.*

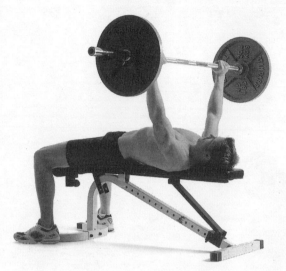

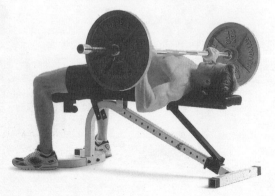

BENCH PRESS

Lie on your back on a flat bench with your feet on the floor. Grab the barbell with an overhand grip, your hands just beyond shoulder-width apart. Lift the bar off the uprights, and hold it at arm's length over your chest. Slowly lower the bar to your chest. Pause, then push the bar back to the starting position.

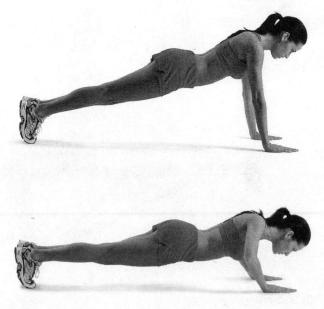

HOME VARIATION: *Just do standard press-ups: get in a press-up position with your hands about shoulder-width apart. Bend at the elbows while keeping your back straight, until your chin almost touches the floor, then push back up.*

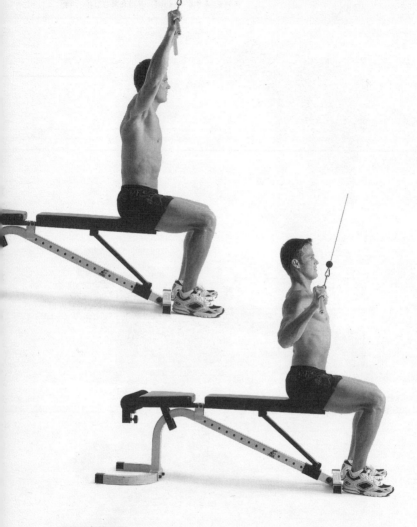

PULLDOWN

Stand facing a lat pulldown machine. Reach up and grasp the bar with an overhand grip that's 10 to 15 cm/ 4 to 6 in wider than your shoulders. Sit on the seat, letting the resistance of the bar extend your arms above your head. When you're in position, pull the bar down until it touches your upper chest. Hold this position for a second, then return to the starting position.

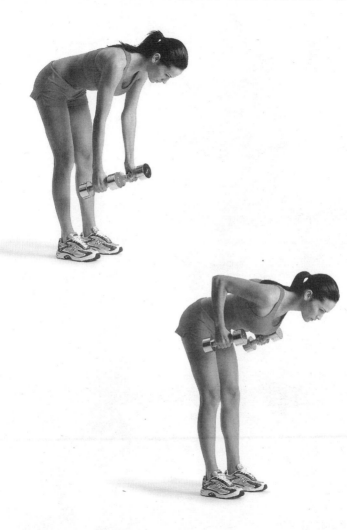

HOME VARIATION: *Bent-Over Row. Stand with your knees slightly bent and shoulder-width apart. Bend over so that your back is almost parallel to the floor. Holding a dumbbell in each hand, let your arms hang towards the floor. With your palms facing in, pull the dumbbells towards you until they touch the outside of your chest. Pause, then return to the starting position.*

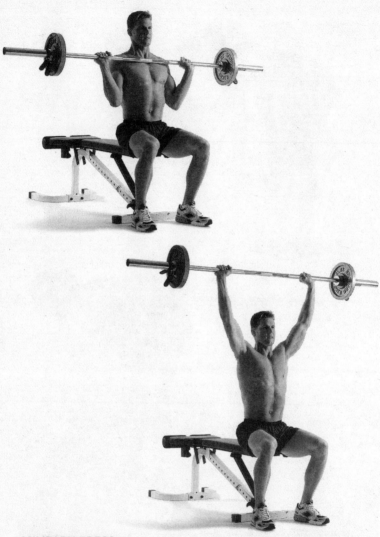

MILITARY PRESS

Sitting on an exercise bench, hold a barbell at shoulder height with your hands shoulder-width apart. Press the weight straight overhead so that your arms are almost fully extended, hold for a count of one, then bring it down to the front of your shoulders. Repeat.

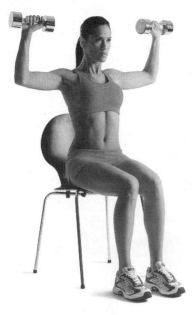

HOME VARIATION: *Sitting on a sturdy chair instead of a bench, hold one dumbbell in each hand, about level with your ears. Push the dumbbells straight overhead so that your arms are almost fully extended, hold for a count of one, then return to the starting position. Repeat.*

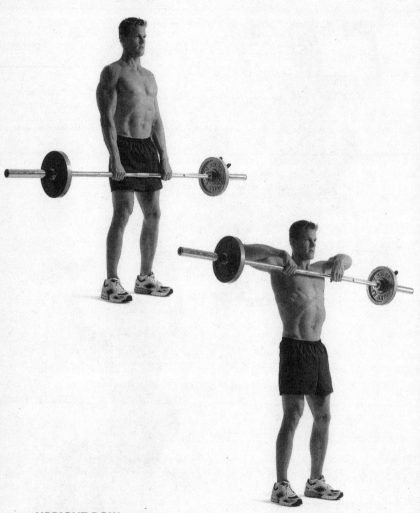

UPRIGHT ROW

Grab a barbell with an overhand grip, and stand with your feet shoulder-width apart and your knees slightly bent. Let the barbell hang at arm's length on top of your thighs, thumbs pointed towards each other. Bending your elbows, lift your upper arms straight out to the sides, and pull the barbell straight up until your upper arms are parallel to the floor and the bar is just below chin level. Pause, then return to the starting position.

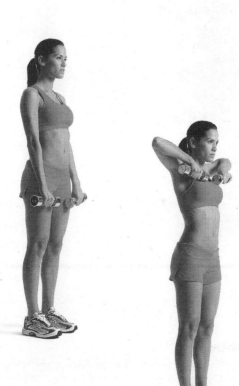

HOME VARIATION: *Same, using one dumbbell in each hand.*

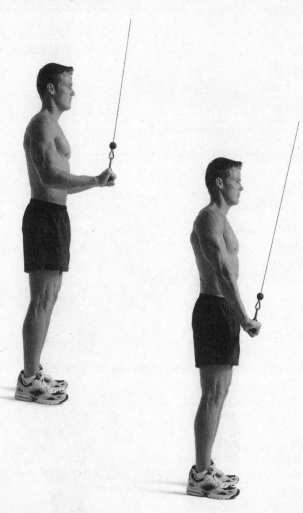

TRICEPS PUSHDOWN

While standing, grip a bar attached to a high pulley cable or lat machine with your hands about 15 cm/ 6 in apart. With your elbows tucked against your sides, bring the bar down until it is directly in front of you. With your fore-arms parallel to the floor (the starting position), push the bar down until your arms are extended straight down with the bar near your thighs. Don't lock your elbows. Return to the starting position.

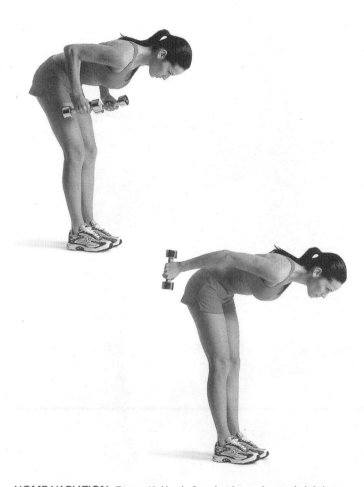

HOME VARIATION: *Triceps Kickback. Stand with your knees slightly bent and shoulder-width apart. Bend over so that your back is almost parallel to the ground. Bend your elbows to about 90-degree angles, raising them to just above the level of your back. This is the starting position. Extend your forearms backwards, keeping your upper arms stationary. When they're fully extended, your arms should be parallel to the ground. Pause, then return to the starting position.*

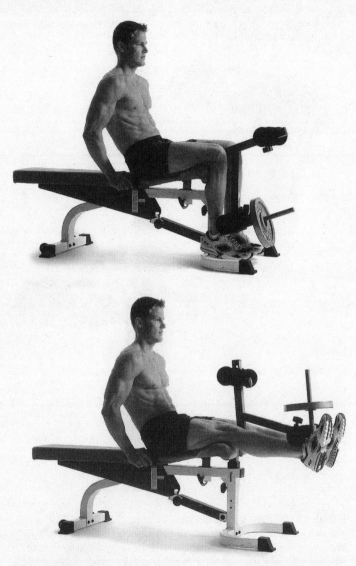

LEG EXTENSION

Sitting on a leg extension machine with your feet under the footpads, lean back slightly, and lift the pads with your feet until your legs are extended.

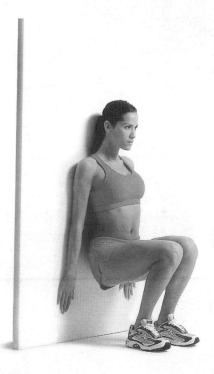

HOME VARIATION: *Squat Against the Wall. Stand with your back flat against a wall. Squat down so that your thighs are parallel to the ground. Hold that position for as long as you can. That consists of one set. Aim for 20 seconds to start, and work your way up to 45 seconds.*

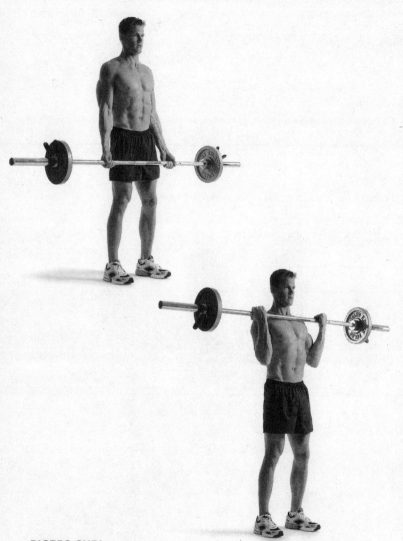

BICEPS CURL

Stand while holding a barbell in front of you, palms facing out, with your hands shoulder-width apart and your arms hanging in front of you. Curl the weight towards your shoulders, hold for a second, then return to the starting position.

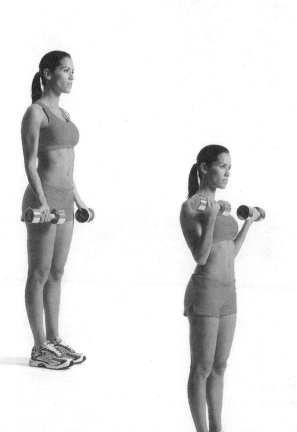

HOME VARIATION: *Same, only use a set of dumbbells instead.*

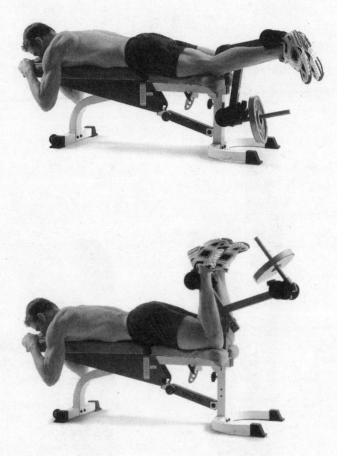

LEG CURL

Lie face-down on a leg curl machine, and hook your ankles under the padded bar. Keeping your stomach and pelvis against the bench, slowly raise your feet towards your buttocks, curling up the weight. Come up so that your feet nearly touch your buttocks, and slowly return to the starting position.

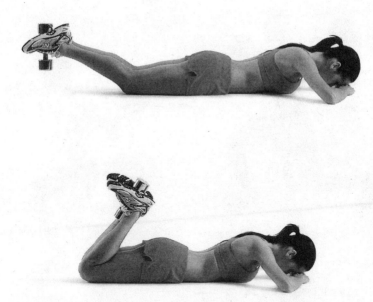

HOME VARIATION: *Lie down with your stomach on the floor. Put a light dumbbell between your feet (so that the top end of the dumbbell rests on the bottom of your feet). Squeeze your feet together, and curl them up towards your buttocks.*

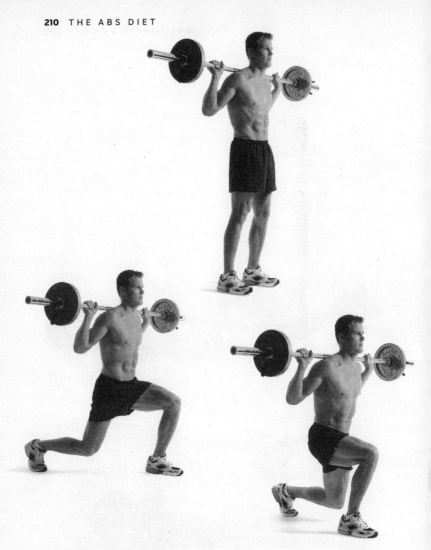

TRAVELLING LUNGE

Rest a barbell across your upper back. Stand, with your feet hip-width apart, at one end of the room; you need room to walk about 20 steps. Step forward with your left foot, and lower your body so that your left thigh is parallel to the floor and your right thigh is perpendicular to the floor (your right knee should bend and almost touch the floor). Stand and bring your right foot up next to your left, then repeat with the right leg lunging forward.

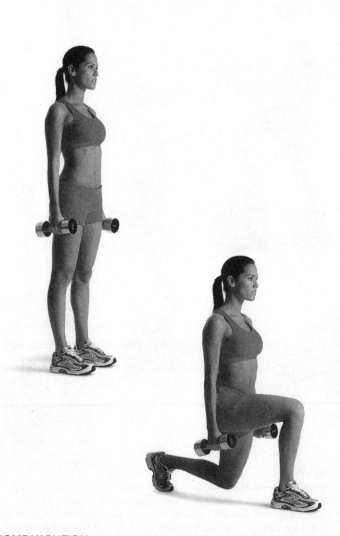

HOME VARIATION: *Use dumbbells, holding one in each hand with your arms at your sides. If you don't have enough space, do the move in one place, alternating your lead foot with each lunge.*

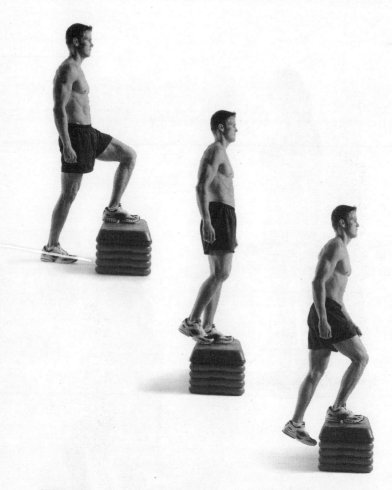

STEP-UP

Use a step or bench that's 45cm/ 18 in off the ground. Place your left foot on the step so that your knee is bent at 90 degrees. Your knee should not advance past the toes of your left foot. Push off with your left foot, and bring your right foot onto the step, keeping your back straight. Now step down with the left foot, followed by the right. Alternate the leading foot, or do all of the repetitions leading with one foot and then alternating. Once you're comfortable, add dumbbells.

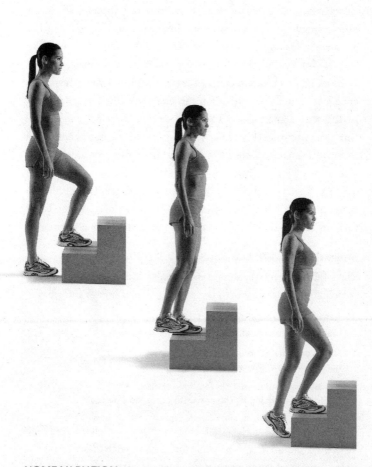

HOME VARIATION: *Same, only use a staircase instead of a step (if you don't have one).*

The Interval Workout

They say that slow and steady wins the race. But the cardiovascular key to fat burning is using interval workouts – workouts that alternate high-intensity levels with lower-intensity effort. As I mentioned earlier, that formula keeps your body burning calories long after you've stopped working out. Interval workouts mimic sports – start-and-stop motions with periods of sprinting or close-to-sprinting speeds followed by light jogging or rest. You can use interval workouts any way you want – running, cycling, swimming, on elliptical trainers, even walking if you alternate a speed walk and slow walk. You can also vary the intensity levels in different combinations. To start, here are three options for setting your workout. (If you use exercise machines, don't choose the interval workout; choose the manual one, and create your own intensities by adjusting it yourself. It'll give you greater control over the speeds and will help you burn fat faster.) You'll derive benefits in as little as a 20-minute interval workout. As you build up endurance and strength, you can add time to your workout.

Interval Variation I: Standard

The following is a typical interval workout. You alternate the same period of low intensity with the same period of higher intensity.

> 3–5 minutes warmup (light jog, low intensity,
> gradually increasing at the end of the warmup period)
>
> 1 minute moderate or high intensity followed
> by 1 minute low intensity (repeat 6–8 times)
>
> 3–5 minutes cooldown (light jog, low intensity,
> gradually decreasing by the end of the cooldown period)

Interval Variation II: Pyramid

This pyramid structure allows you to start with short bursts of speed, and then you'll peak at the longest surge of energy in the middle of your workout before coming back down.

3–5 minutes warmup

30 seconds high intensity

1 minute low intensity

45 seconds high intensity

1 minute low intensity

60 seconds high intensity

1 minute low intensity

90 seconds high intensity

1 minute low intensity

60 seconds high intensity

1 minute low intensity

45 seconds high intensity

1 minute low intensity

30 seconds high intensity

3–5 minutes cooldown

Interval Variation III: Sports Conditioning

Sports are unpredictable. This interval workout simulates some of that unpredictability by having you doing different times and different intensities. You can mix and match the orders and repetitions as much as you want. Rest longer after the periods in which you use the most energy.

3–5 minutes warmup

2 minutes moderate or high intensity followed
by 2 minutes low intensity (repeat once)

30 seconds high intensity followed by 30 seconds low intensity
(repeat four times)

60-metre sprints (or 10 seconds if not running)
followed by 90 seconds rest (repeat 6–10 times)

3–5 minutes cooldown

Chapter 13

TARGETING YOUR ABS

A '56-Pack' of Exercises

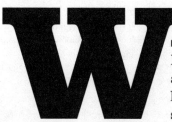**HEN I WAS IN COLLEGE,** I had a friend who argued that he knew the key to a six-pack: 'All you have to do is 1,000 crunches a day for a month.' He said it in a way that made you believe him – that if only you were disciplined enough to put in the time every day to concentrate on your abdominal muscles, then you'd eventually chisel away a gut of stone. His theory was that it all boiled down to volume and discipline. He went on to say that the iconic ab exercise would do more than just build abs – that it was also the fix-all to weight problems, that you could simply crunch away years of bingeing on pizza, burgers and all-night boozing.

In a lot of ways (a heck of a lot of ways, actually), my friend was wrong. For one, crunching won't burn fat. And you won't develop abs by doing the same exercise over and over – let alone the same exercise every day. And 1,000 repetitions? C'mon. There's only one thing most of us would do 1,000 times a day if it were physically possible, and it wouldn't be a crunch. But he was right in one sense: if you want abs that will make you stronger, healthier and better looking, you do have to work them. And that does take discipline – but not as much as you'd think.

Though your midsection works as one unified core, it does help to think of your abdominal centre in regions. To build speed-bump abs, you need to work the entire region. The three visible regions

REACQUAINT YOURSELF WITH YOUR ABS

Your abdominal muscles are a lot like a skilled group of employees. The harder they work, the better they make you look, and vice versa.

This is because you use your abs in virtually every movement that matters. Lifting. Running. Jumping. Reproducing. (It takes a lot of midsection stability to stand over that copy machine. Especially when it's printing on both sides of the page.) So the stronger they are, the harder and longer you'll be able to play. Here's a quick course in the anatomy of your abs.

Rectus abdominis. This is the six-pack muscle that helps your upper body bend (like in a crunch) and also helps keep good posture. It's what people think of when they think of abs.

External obliques. These muscles start on the ribs and extend diagonally down the sides of your waist. If a movement happens at your waist, the external obliques are involved. The torso rotation that's key to golf, tennis and hockey is mostly a function of the external obliques. Even the basic crunching motion, attributed to the rectus abdominis (the six-pack muscle), wouldn't be possible without a strong contraction of the external obliques to stabilize the torso.

Internal obliques. These lie between the rib cage and the external obliques, and also extend diagonally down the sides of your waist. Similar to the externals, the internal obliques are involved in torso rotation. You use these muscles when you breathe deeply.

Transverse abdominis. It's a thin muscle that runs horizontally, surrounding your abdomen. It's also known as 'the girdle' because it functions as a compressor for the abdomen, keeping everything in place.

consist of the upper abs, the lower abs and the obliques (the muscles along the side of your torso). But there are also a number of supporting muscles that, when developed, will add strength to your abdominals: your lower back and the transverse abdominis – muscles that run underneath your abdomen horizontally to give support to your entire midsection.

You already have all of these muscles; you just need to break them out. That's why your priorities have to revolve around the first two components: the nutrition principles and the fat-burning workout. Once you strip away the fat, your abs can grow and show. Unlike what my friend said, you won't get a six-pack by working your abdominal muscles every day. Instead, follow these guidelines for adding the final component.

Work your abs 2 or 3 days a week. Abs are like any other muscle in your body. They'll grow when they're at rest, not when you're working them. So working them every day doesn't give them a chance to grow and get strong. You will develop abs by working them two or three times a week. I'd recommend adding the ab circuit to the beginning of your workout. Saving them until the end means there's more chance that you'll skimp and take shortcuts.

Hit the whole region. You have five regions of your abdominals that you're going to work. For each workout, pick one exercise per region to ensure that you're hitting every area.

Pick different exercises every workout. We're giving you 56 different exercises for your abdominals, but you need to pick only five exercises each workout. The key is variety: changing your routine doesn't allow your abs to get comfortable, so they'll continue to grow after each workout.

Do a circuit. In the first week of workouts, just do one set of each exercise (10 to 15 repetitions, depending on the exercise). In the second and third week, do two sets if you'd like, but perform them in a circuit so that you're doing each exercise once before repeating an exercise. After that, you can do three circuits. Even then, your ab workouts shouldn't take more than 5 minutes.

Go slow. Each rep of an ab exercise should last slightly longer than you lasted on your first date – 4 to 6 seconds. Any faster, and you run the risk of letting momentum do the work. The slower you go, the higher the intensity. The higher the intensity, the stronger the stomach.

In this chapter, you'll find 56 exercises – a '56-pack' of exercises – so that you'll never get bored and so that you'll work your abdominals as efficiently as possible. Remember that this portion of the workout is what will make your abs pop out of your skin the way Lady Gaga pops out of her wardrobe. Think of the ab exercise portion of the plan as the toy at the bottom of the cereal box, the pay cheque at the end of the month, the finish line at the end of the marathon. It's the motivation. It's the reward. It's the goal that no scales could ever show.

How to Do the Workout

PICK ONE EXERCISE from each group of the listings below, and do the exercise for the specified number of repetitions. Do one set of each exercise, and then repeat the circuit.

Note: Many of these exercises target different regions of the abdominals during the same movement, but they're grouped based on what areas they primarily target. They've also been grouped by levels of difficulty so that you can change your workouts as you get stronger. For each exercise, pause at the end of the movement, and return to the starting position. That counts as one repetition, unless otherwise noted.

The Abs Circuit

Upper Abs

Lower Abs

Obliques

Transverse Abdominis

Lower Back

Upper Abs

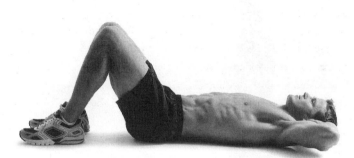

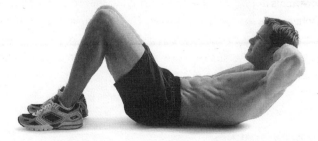

TRADITIONAL CRUNCH

Lie on your back with your knees bent and your hands behind your ears.
Slowly crunch up, bringing your shoulder blades off the ground.

12–15 repetitions [Beginner]

Upper Abs

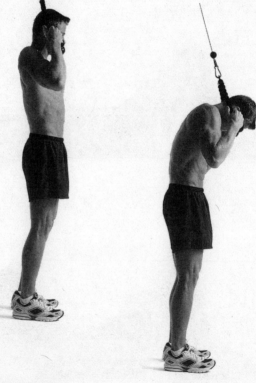

STANDING CRUNCH

Attach a rope handle to a high cable pulley. Stand with your back to the weight stack, and hold the ends of the rope behind your head. Crunch down.

12–15 repetitions [*Beginner*]

Upper Abs

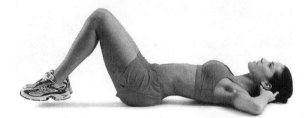

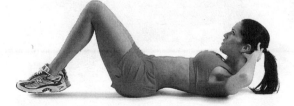

MODIFIED RAISED-FEET CRUNCHES

Lie on your back with your knees bent and your hands behind your ears.
Raise your feet just a few centimetres/inches off the floor, and hold them
there. Crunch up, then lower your torso back to the floor, keeping your feet
raised throughout the movement.

12–15 repetitions [*Beginner to intermediate*]

Upper Abs

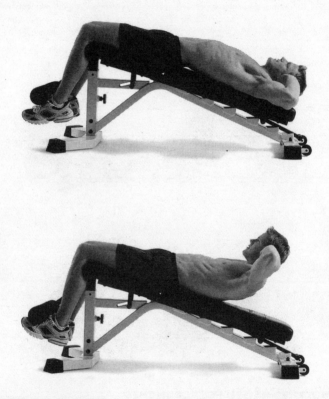

DECLINE CRUNCH

Lie on your back on a decline board, with your ankles locked under the padded support bars and your fingertips cupped behind your ears. Lift your shoulder blades off the bench, keeping your lower body flat. Don't jerk your body to build momentum. Hold the contraction for a second.

12–15 repetitions [*Beginner to intermediate*]

Upper Abs

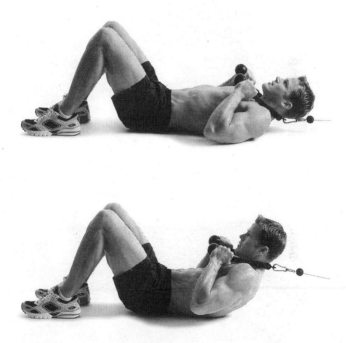

LYING CABLE CRUNCH

Attach a rope handle to the low pulley. Lie on the floor with your head near the low pulley, your knees bent, and your feet flat on the floor. Hold the handle over your chest so that the point of the rope attachment is at the base of your neck. Crunch your rib cage towards your pelvis, lifting your shoulder blades a few centimetres/inches off the floor.

12–15 repetitions [*Intermediate to advanced*]

Upper Abs

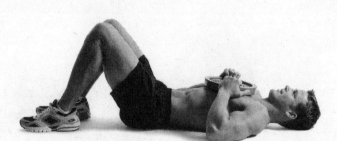

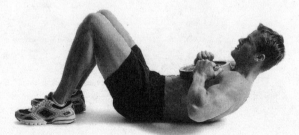

WEIGHTED CRUNCH

Lie on your back with your knees bent, holding a weight plate or dumbbell across your chest. Slowly crunch up, bringing your shoulder blades off the ground. Use progressively heavier weight.

12–15 repetitions [Intermediate to advanced]

Upper Abs

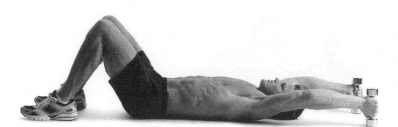

LONG-ARM WEIGHTED CRUNCH

Lie on your back with your knees bent. Hold a light dumbbell in each hand, and stretch your arms straight back behind you. Crunch your rib cage towards your pelvis. Don't generate momentum with your arms.

12–15 repetitions [*Intermediate to advanced*]

Upper Abs

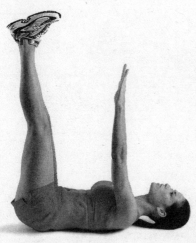

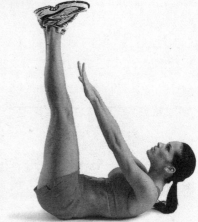

TOE TOUCH

Lie on your back with your legs raised directly over your hips; your knees should be slightly bent. Raise your arms straight up, pointing towards your toes, and relax your head and neck. Use your upper abs to raise your rib cage towards your pelvis, lift your shoulder blades off the floor, and reach towards your toes. Hold for a second. Lower your shoulders to the floor and repeat.

12–15 repetitions [*Intermediate to advanced*]

Upper Abs

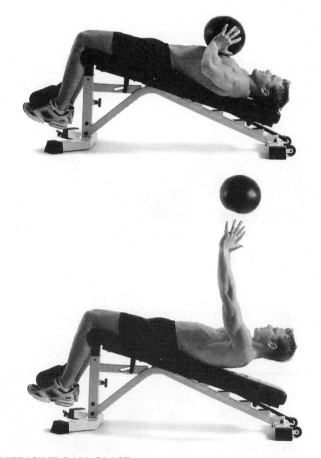

MEDICINE BALL BLAST

Set an adjustable ab bench at a 45-degree angle. Lie down on it with your head towards the floor, and hook your feet under the padded support bars. Hold a medicine ball at your chest as you lower yourself. As you come up, chest-pass the ball straight up over your head. Catch it at the top of the movement, then lower yourself and repeat.

12–15 repetitions [*Advanced*]

Upper Abs

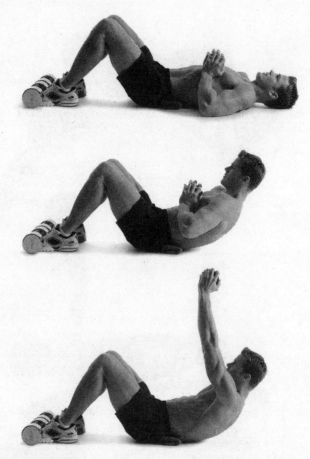

SICILIAN CRUNCH

Slide your feet under the handles of heavy dumbbells. Place a rolled-up towel under your lower back, and hold a dumbbell across your chest. Raise your upper body as high as possible by crunching your rib cage towards your pelvis. At the top of the move, straighten your arms and raise the dumbbell above your head. Keep the dumbbell above your head, and take 4 seconds to lower your body to the starting position.

10 repetitions [*Advanced*]

Lower Abs

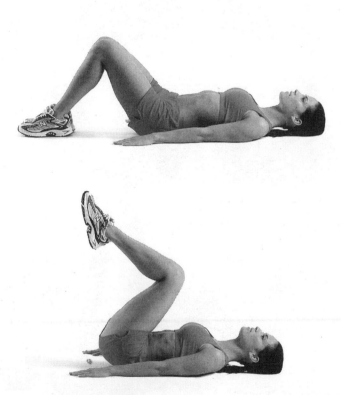

BENT-LEG KNEE RAISE

Lie on your back with your head and neck relaxed and your hands on the
floor near your buttocks. Your feet should be flat on the floor. Use your lower
abdominal muscles to raise your knees up towards your rib cage, then slowly
lower your feet back to the starting position. As your feet lightly touch the
floor, repeat.

12 repetitions [*Beginner*]

Lower Abs

PULSE-UP

Lie with your hands underneath your tailbone and your
legs raised and pointed straight up towards the ceiling, perpendicular to
your torso. Pull your navel inwards, and flex your glutes as you lift your hips
just a few centimetres/inches off the floor. Then lower your hips.

12 repetitions [*Beginner*]

Lower Abs

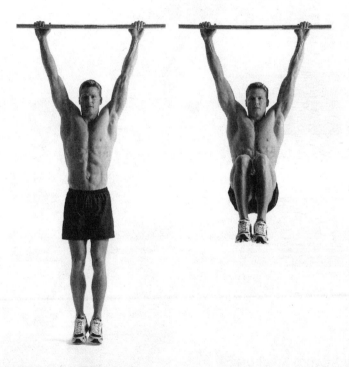

HANGING KNEE RAISE

Hang fully extended from a chin-up bar, with your palms facing out and your hands a little further than shoulder-width apart. (Your feet may lightly touch the floor.) Raise your knees towards your chest, curling your pelvis upwards at the end. When you can do that for 12 repetitions, make it tougher by keeping your legs straight instead of bending your knees or by holding a medicine ball between your knees.

12 repetitions [*Beginner to intermediate*]

Lower Abs

SEATED AB CRUNCH

Sit on the edge of a stable chair or bench. Place your hands in front of your buttocks, and grip the sides of the seat. Lean back slightly and extend your legs down and away, keeping your heels 10 to 15cm/4 to 6 in off the floor. To begin the exercise, bend your knees and slowly raise your legs towards your chest. At the same time, lean forward with your upper body, allowing your chest to approach your thighs.

12 repetitions [*Beginner to intermediate*]

Lower Abs

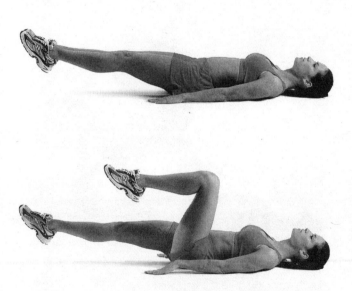

RAISED KNEE-IN

Lie on your back. Your arms should be close to your sides, with your palms down and just under your lower back and buttocks. Press the small of your back against the floor, and extend your legs outwards, with your heels about 8 cm/3 in above the floor. Keeping your lower back against the floor, lift your left knee towards your chest. Your right leg should remain hovering above the floor. Hold, then straighten your left leg to the starting position and repeat with your right leg. Keep your abs tight throughout the exercise.

8–12 repetitions each side [*Intermediate*]

Lower Abs

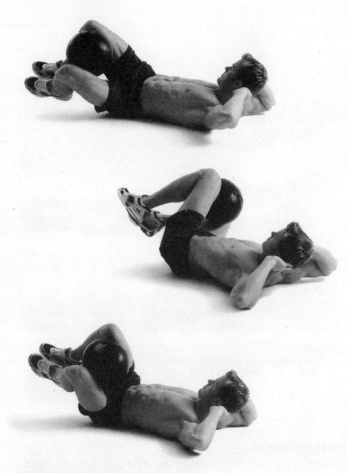

FIGURE-8 CRUNCH

Lie on your back with your knees bent at a 90-degree angle and your feet flat on the floor. Squeeze a light medicine ball tightly between your knees. Cup your hands lightly over your ears, then slowly raise your head, shoulders and feet off the floor. Move your knees in a wide figure-of-eight motion.
Do 3 repetitions in one direction, then reverse the motion for 3 repetitions.

6 repetitions [Intermediate]

Lower Abs

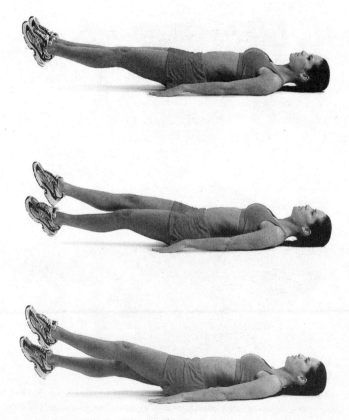

FLUTTER KICK
Lie on your back, raise both feet about 30 cm/1 ft off the ground, and scissor-kick one leg over the other.

20 repetitions [*Intermediate*]

Lower Abs

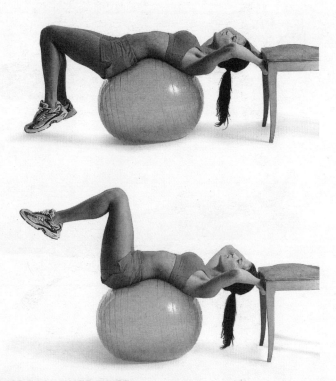

SWISS BALL KNEE RAISE

Lie face-up on a Swiss ball, with your hips lower than your shoulders. Reach back and grab something that won't move, such as a bench or desk. Lift and bend your legs so that your feet are off the floor and the lower parts of your legs point ahead. (To make it more difficult, hold your legs straight out.) Do a standard Bent-Leg Knee Raise, using your abs and hip flexors to curl your knees towards your chest.

12 repetitions [*Intermediate to advanced*]

Lower Abs

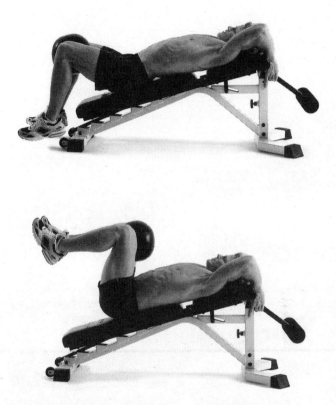

REVERSE CRUNCH HOLDING MEDICINE BALL

Lie on a slant board with your hips lower than your head. Grab the bar behind your head for support. Bend your hips and knees at 90-degree angles, and hold a small medicine ball between your knees. Start with your buttocks flat against the board. Pull your hips up and in towards your rib cage. Curl them as high as you can without lifting your shoulders off the board, and keep your hips and knees at 90-degree angles.

12 repetitions [*Intermediate to advanced*]

Lower Abs

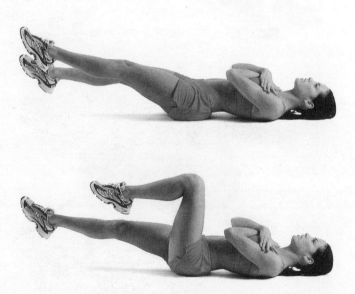

PUSH-AWAYS

Lie on your back with your hands on your chest, legs extended, feet raised off the floor. Alternately bring each knee towards your head, then forcefully kick forwards. Don't let your feet touch the floor. (If you feel any discomfort in your lower back while performing this exercise, try lifting your head and tucking your chin towards your chest.)

10 repetitions each side [*Intermediate to advanced*]

Obliques

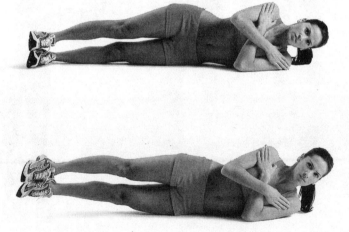

OBLIQUE V-UP

Lie on your side with your body in a straight line. Fold your arms across your chest. Keeping your legs together, lift them off the floor as you raise your top elbow towards your hip. The range of motion is short, but you should feel an intense contraction in your obliques.

10 repetitions each side [Beginner]

Obliques

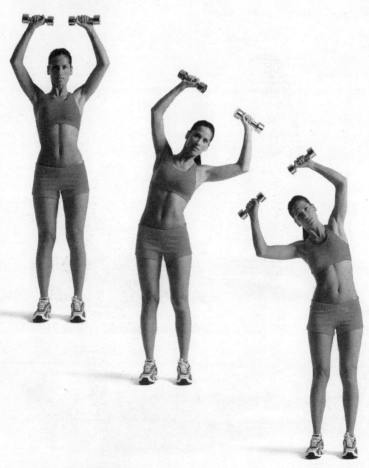

SAXON SIDE BEND

Hold a pair of lightweight dumbbells over your head, in line with your shoulders, with your elbows slightly bent. Keep your back straight, and slowly bend directly to your left side as far as possible without twisting your upper body. Pause, return to an upright position, then bend to your right side as far as possible.

6–10 repetitions on each side [*Beginner to intermediate*]

Obliques

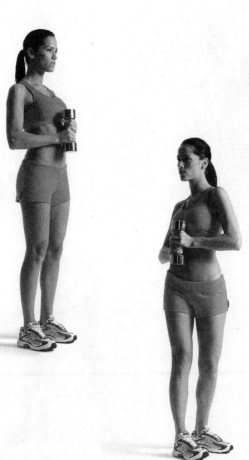

SPEED ROTATION

Stand while holding a dumbbell with both hands in front of your midsection. Twist 90 degrees to the right, then 180 degrees to your left. Keep your abs tight and move fast. Bring to the centre. Alternate the side you start with.

10 repetitions each side [*Intermediate*]

Obliques

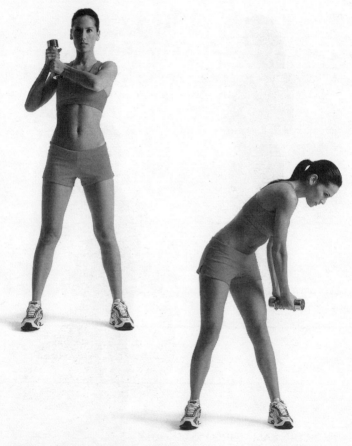

TWO-HANDED WOOD CHOP

Stand while holding a dumbbell, with both hands next to your right ear.
Flex your abs and rotate your torso to the left as you extend your arms
and lower the dumbbell to the outside of your left knee. Lift it back, finish
the set, and repeat on the other side.

10 repetitions each side *[Intermediate]*

Obliques

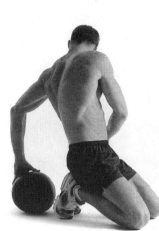

MEDICINE BALL TORSO ROTATION

Hold a medicine ball or basketball in front of you. Sit with your knees bent and your feet on the floor. Quickly twist to your left, and set the ball behind your back. Twist to the right, and pick up the ball. Bring the ball around to your left, and set it down again. Repeat. Do the same number of repetitions in which you first twist to the left side as you do when you twist to the right side.

10 repetitions each side [Intermediate to advanced]

Obliques

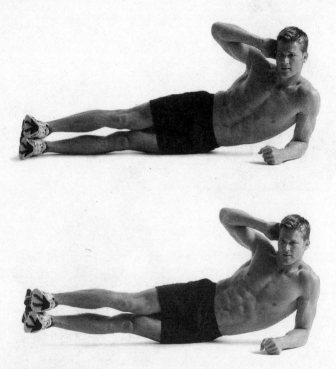

SIDE JACKKNIFE

Lie on your left hip, with your legs nearly straight and slightly raised off the floor. Also raise your torso off the floor, with your left forearm on the floor for balance. Hold your other hand behind your right ear, with your elbow pointed towards your feet. Lift your legs towards your torso while keeping your torso stationary. Pause to feel the contraction on the right side of your waist. Then slowly lower your legs and repeat. Finish the set on that side, then lie on your right hip and do the same number of repetitions.

10 repetitions each side [*Intermediate to advanced*]

Transverse Abdominis

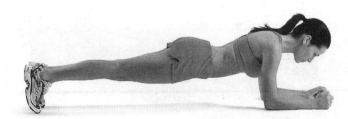

BRIDGE

Start to get in a press-up position, but bend your elbows and rest your weight on your forearms instead of your hands. Your body should form a straight line from your shoulders to your ankles. Pull your abdominals in; imagine you're trying to move your tummy button back to your spine. Hold for 20 seconds, breathing steadily. As you build endurance, you can do one 60-second set.

1–2 repetitions [*Beginner to intermediate*]

Transverse Abdominis

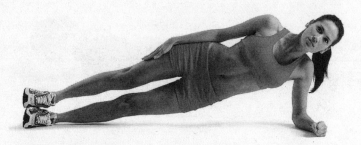

SIDE BRIDGE

Lie on your non-dominant side. Support your weight with that forearm and the outside edge of that foot. Your body should form a straight line from head to ankles. Pull your abs in as far as you can, and hold this position for 10 to 30 seconds, breathing steadily. Relax. If you can do 30 seconds, do one repetition. If not, try for any combination of reps that gets you up to 30 seconds. Repeat on your other side.

1–2 repetitions on each side [*Beginner to intermediate*]

Transverse Abdominis

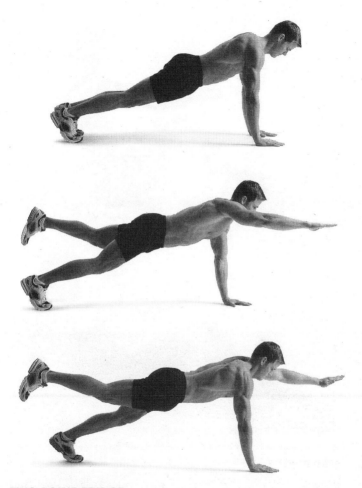

TWO-POINT BRIDGE

Get into the standard press-up position. Lift your right arm and your left leg off the floor at the same time. Hold for 3 to 5 seconds. That's one repetition. Return to the starting position, then repeat, lifting your left arm and right leg this time.

6–10 repetitions each side *[Intermediate]*

Transverse Abdominis

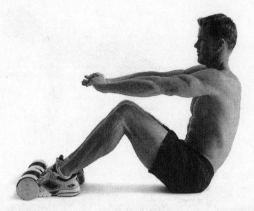

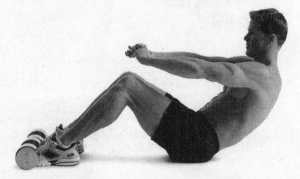

NEGATIVE CRUNCH

Sit on the floor with your knees bent and your feet flat on the floor and shoulder-width apart. Extend your arms with your fingers interlaced, palms facing your knees. Begin with your upper body at slightly less than a 90-degree angle to the floor. Lower your body towards the floor, curling your torso forward, rounding your lower back, and keeping your abs contracted. When your body reaches a 45-degree angle to the floor, return to the starting position. (*Note:* You may need to tuck your feet under a set of weights to help maintain balance throughout the exercise.)

10 repetitions [*Intermediate*]

Transverse Abdominis

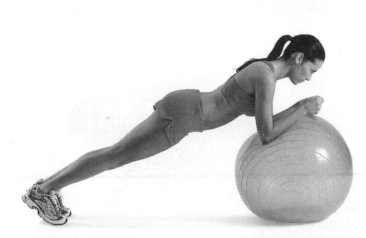

SWISS BALL BRIDGE

Rest your forearms on the ball and your toes on the floor, with your body in a straight line. Pull your stomach in, trying to bring your tummy button to your spine. Hold for 20 seconds, breathing steadily. As you build endurance, you can do one 60-second set.

1–2 repetitions [*Intermediate to advanced*]

Transverse Abdominis

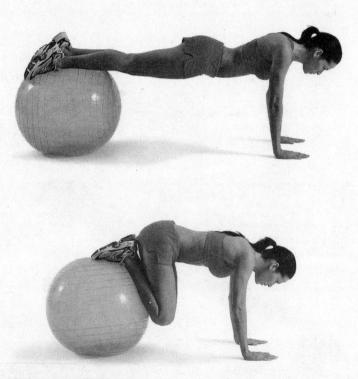

SWISS BALL PULL-INS

Get into the press-up position – your hands set slightly wider than and in line with your shoulders – but instead of placing your feet on the floor, rest your shins on a Swiss ball. With your arms straight and your back flat, your body should form a straight line from your shoulders to your ankles. Roll the Swiss ball towards your chest. Pause, then return the ball to the starting position by extending your legs to the starting position and rolling the ball backwards.

5–10 repetitions [*Intermediate to advanced*]

Transverse Abdominis

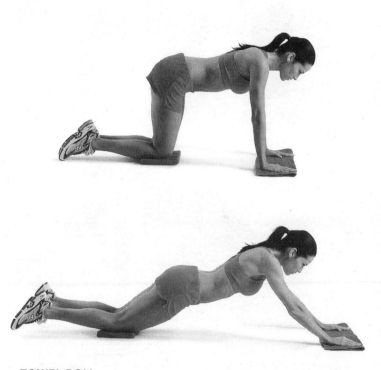

TOWEL ROLL

Kneel on a towel or mat on a tile or wooden floor. Put a towel on the floor in front of you, and place your hands on it. Slide the towel across the floor until your body is fully extended. Your body should look as if you're in a diving position. Slowly slide back up.

5–10 repetitions [*Advanced*]

Transverse Abdominis

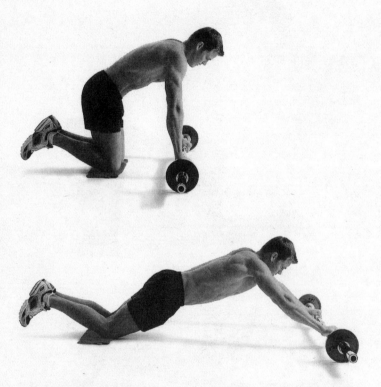

BARBELL ROLLOUT

Load a pair of 2.25-kg/5-lb plates into a barbell. Kneel on an exercise mat or
towel, with your shoulders directly over the bar. Grab the bar with an overhand, shoulder-width grip. Start with your back in a slightly rounded position,
allowing it to extend into a more neutral position as you execute the movement. Roll the bar out in front of you, holding your knees in place as your
hips, torso and arms go forward. Keeping your arms taut, advance as far as
you can without arching your back or touching the floor with anything above
your knees. Pause for a split second, then pull back to the starting position.

5–10 repetitions [Advanced]

Lower Back

BACK EXTENSION

Position yourself in a back extension station, and hook your feet under the leg anchor. Hold your arms straight out in front of you. Your body should form a straight line from your hands to your hips. Lower your torso, allowing your lower back to round, until it's just short of perpendicular to the floor. Raise your upper body until it's slightly above parallel to the floor. At this point, you should have a slight arch in your back, and your shoulder blades should be pulled together. Pause for a second, then repeat.

12–15 repetitions [*Beginner to intermediate*]

Lower Back

TWISTING BACK EXTENSION

Position yourself in a back extension station, and hook your feet under the leg anchor. Place your fingers lightly behind or over your ears. Lower your upper body, allowing your lower back to round, until it's just short of perpendicular to the floor. Raise and twist your upper body until it's slightly above parallel to the floor and facing left. Pause, then lower your torso and repeat, this time twisting to the right.

12–15 repetitions [Intermediate]

Lower Back

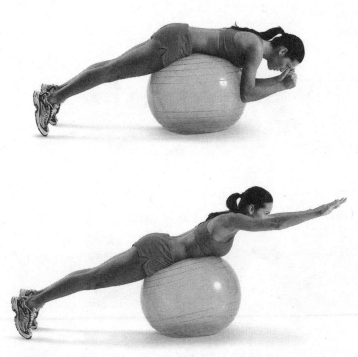

SWISS BALL SUPERMAN

Lie face-down over a Swiss ball so that your hips are pressed against the ball and your torso is rounded over it. Lift your upper arms so that they're parallel to your body, and bend your elbows 90 degrees so that your fingers are pointing forward and your elbows are pointing back. Slowly extend your back until your chest is completely off the ball, extend your arms forward, and hold that position. Draw your arms back into position as you return your torso to the ball.

12–15 repetitions [Intermediate]

Lower Back

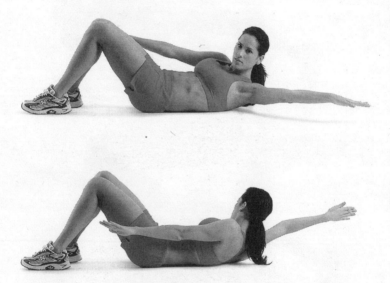

SWIMMER'S BACKSTROKE

Lie face-up on the floor, with your knees bent and feet flat. Flatten your lower back against the floor. Now do a crunch to flex your trunk forward, and lift your shoulder blades as high off the floor as you possibly can. Keeping your chest high, perform a backstroke with one arm at a time, allowing your torso to twist towards the arm that's reaching back. Work up to 5 repetitions of 45 seconds each, alternating arms. The higher you lift your chest off the floor, the better your exercise will work. Add light dumbbells when the move becomes too easy.

1–5 repetitions [*Intermediate to advanced*]

BONUS! THE 18 ABOVE-THE-BELT TIME SAVERS!

Looking to shave even more time off your workout while shaving fat from your waistline? The remaining 18 moves of our '56-pack' plan work several areas of your midsection simultaneously. Use any one of the following substitutions to cover two or three areas with one exercise, and you can reduce your workout plan to just a few exercises instead of five!

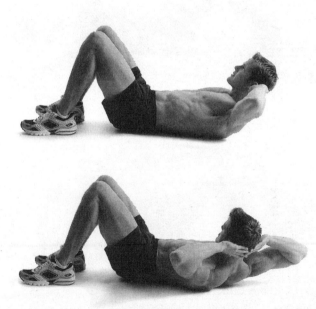

CRUNCH/SIDE BEND COMBO
Targets both the upper abs and obliques

Lie on your back, with your knees bent and your hands behind your ears. Curl up so that your shoulder blades are off the floor. Bend at the waist to the left, aiming your left armpit towards your right hip. Straighten, then bend to your right.

8 repetitions to each side [*Beginner*]

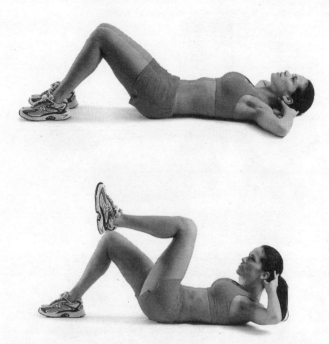

SINGLE-KNEE CRUNCH
Targets both the upper and lower abs

Lie on your back, with your hips bent 90 degrees and your feet flat on the floor. Touch your fingers to the sides of your head, with your elbows bent. Raise your head, shoulders and buttocks off the floor as you simultaneously bring your left knee towards your chest. Lower your torso and leg back down, then repeat the exercise, this time drawing your right knee up instead as you crunch.

10 repetitions each side [*Beginner to intermediate*]

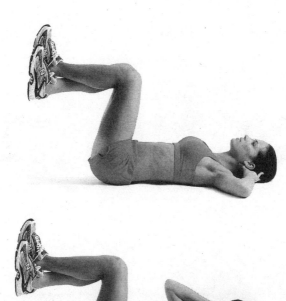

TWISTING CRUNCH
Targets both the upper abs and obliques

Lie on your back on the floor, with your hands cupped behind your ears and your elbows out. Cross your ankles, with your knees slightly bent, and raise your legs until your thighs are perpendicular to your body. Bring your right shoulder off the floor as you cross your right elbow over to your left knee. Return to the starting position and repeat, beginning with the left shoulder, crossing your left elbow over to your right knee.

8 repetitions to each side [*Beginner to intermediate*]

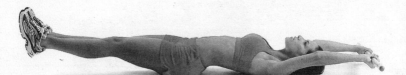

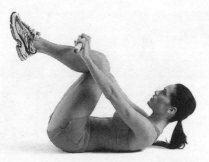

STICK CRUNCH
Targets both the upper and lower abs

Lie on your back, with your feet raised off the ground and your knees slightly bent. Hold a broomstick behind your head, with your arms extended and off the ground. Crunch your torso up, and draw your knees up so that the stick extends past your knees. Pause, then return to the starting position.

12 repetitions [*Intermediate*]

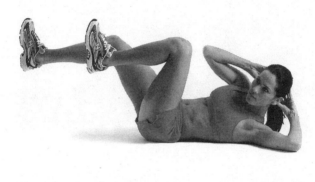

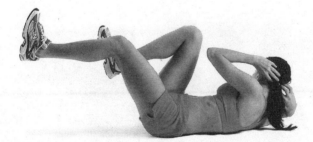

BICYCLE
Targets both the upper and lower abs

Lying on your back with your knees bent 90 degrees and your hands behind your ears, pump your legs back and forth, bicycle-style, as you rotate your torso from side to side by moving an armpit (not an elbow) towards the opposite knee.

20 repetitions [*Intermediate*]

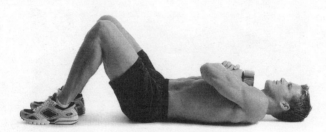

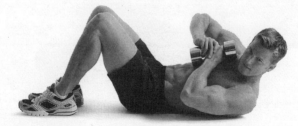

WEIGHTED ONE-SIDED CRUNCH
Targets both the upper abs and obliques

Lie with your knees bent and feet flat on the floor. Hold a dumbbell by
your right shoulder with both hands. Curl your torso up and rotate to the left.
Lower yourself, finish the set, then repeat, placing the dumbbell next to your
left shoulder.

8 repetitions to each side [*Intermediate*]

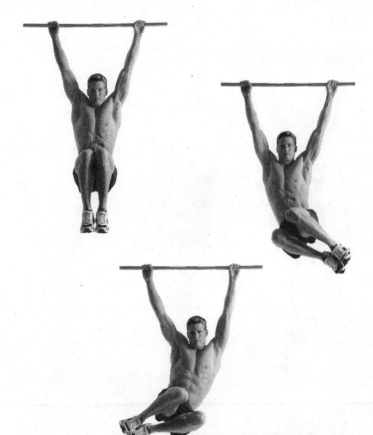

OBLIQUE HANGING LEG RAISE
Targets both the lower abs and obliques

Grasp a chin-up bar with an overhand grip and hang from it at arm's length, with your knees bent. Keep your knees bent, and lift your left hip towards your left armpit until your lower legs are nearly parallel to the floor. Pause, then return to the starting position, and lift your right hip towards your right armpit.

10 repetitions each side [*Intermediate*]

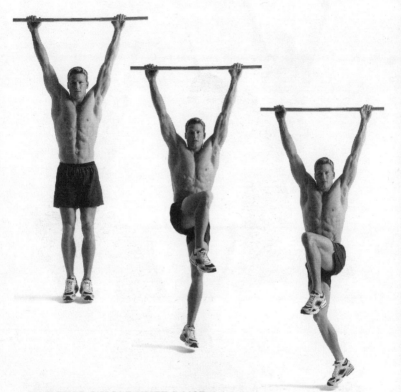

HANGING SINGLE-KNEE RAISE
Targets both the lower abs and obliques

Hang fully extended from a chin-up bar, with your palms facing out and your hands a little further than shoulder-width apart. Your feet should lightly touch the floor. Without swinging to pick up momentum, raise your right knee towards your left shoulder as far as you can, using your abs for power. Slightly thrust your pelvis forward to help, but don't rock. Hold for a second, then lower to the starting position. Repeat with your left leg, raising it towards your right shoulder.

8–12 repetitions each side [Intermediate]

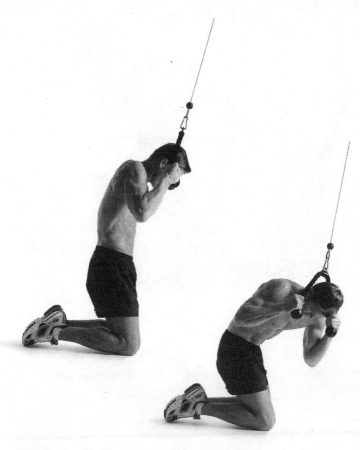

KNEELING THREE-WAY CABLE CRUNCH
Targets both the upper abs and obliques

Attach a rope to the handle of the high pulley. Kneel facing the pulley,
and grab the ends of the rope, with your palms facing each other. Hold
the rope along the sides of your face, with your elbows slightly bent.
Bend forward at the waist, rounding your back and aiming your chest at your
pelvis. Stop when you feel a contraction in your abdominal muscles. Return to
the starting position, then repeat the movement, this time aiming your chest
towards your left knee. Stop when you feel a contraction in your left obliques.
Return, then repeat the movement to your right. That's one repetition.

8 repetitions [Intermediate to advanced]

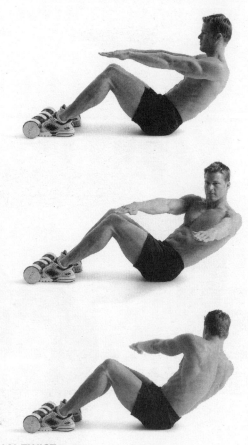

RUSSIAN TWIST
Targets both the upper abs and obliques

Sit on the floor, with your knees bent and your feet flat. Hold your arms straight out in front of your chest, with your palms facing down. Lean back so that your torso is at a 45-degree angle to the floor. Twist to the left as far as you can, pause, then reverse your movement and twist all the way back to the right as far as you can. As you get stronger, hold a light weight in your hands as you do the movement. (*Note:* You may need to tuck your feet under a set of weights to help maintain balance throughout the exercise.)

10 repetitions each side [*Intermediate to advanced*]

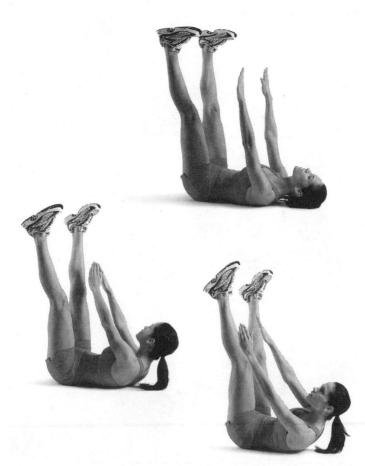

V-SPREAD TOE TOUCH
Targets both the upper abs and obliques

Lie flat on your back, with your legs straight up in a V position without locking your knees. Raise your arms towards the ceiling. Curl your shoulder blades up, and reach towards your right foot with both hands. Hold for a second, concentrating on your abs, then lower to the starting position. Repeat, this time reaching for your left foot. Don't pause at the lower position.

12–15 repetitions [*Intermediate to advanced*]

CORKSCREW
Targets both the lower abs and obliques

Lie on your back, with your legs raised directly over your hips; your knees
should be slightly bent. Place your hands with the palms down at your sides.
Use your lower abs to raise your hips off the floor and towards your rib cage,
elevating your hips straight up towards the ceiling. Simultaneously twist your
hips to the right in a corkscrew motion. Hold, then return to the starting
position. Repeat, twisting to the left.

10 repetitions [Intermediate to advanced]

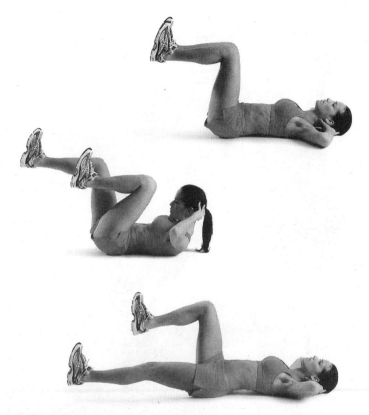

STRAIGHT-LEG CYCLING CRUNCH
Targets both the upper and lower abs

Lie on your back, and bend your hips and knees 90 degrees so that your feet are in the air. Place your hands behind your ears, and perform an abdominal crunch by lifting your head and shoulders off the floor. At the same time, lift your left leg to your chest. Lower your torso to the floor as you straighten your left leg, keeping it a few centimetres/inches off the floor. Repeat the exercise, this time drawing your right knee up as you crunch. Alternate from left to right throughout the exercise.

10 repetitions each side [*Advanced*]

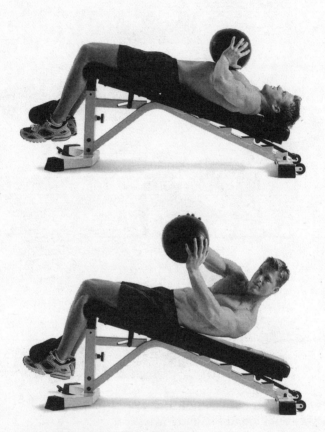

LATERAL MEDICINE BALL BLAST
Targets both the upper abs and obliques
Set an adjustable ab bench at a 45-degree angle. Lie down on it, and hook your feet under the padded support bars. Hold a medicine ball or weight plate against your chest. As you come up, twist to the left and extend your arms as if you were throwing the ball or weight. Pull it back to your chest as you untwist and lower yourself. Repeat, twisting to the right.

5 repetitions each side [Advanced]

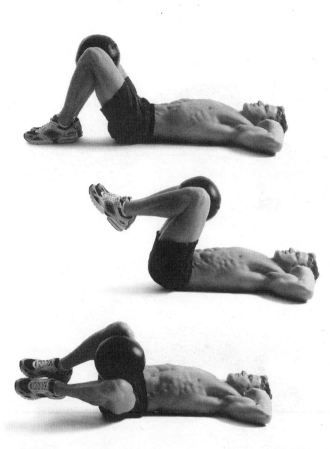

KNEE RAISE WITH DROP
Targets both the lower abs and obliques

Lie on your back, with your hands behind your ears, hips and knees bent, and feet on the floor. Position a medicine ball between your knees. Keep your lower back on the floor throughout the exercise. Contract your abdominals, and pull your knees to your chest. Lower your knees to the left, bring them back to the centre, then return to the starting position. Drop your knees to the right on the next repetition, and alternate sides for each rep.

12 repetitions *[Advanced]*

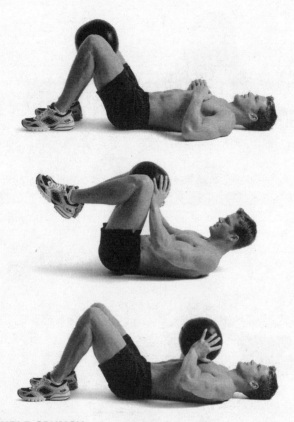

DOUBLE CRUNCH
Targets both the upper and lower abs

Lie on your back, with your hips and knees bent and your feet on the floor. Rest your hands lightly on your chest. Position a medicine ball between your knees. Exhale as you lift your shoulders off the floor and bring your knees to your chest. Grab the ball with your hands, and bring it to your chest as you inhale and return your shoulders and legs to the starting position. Transfer the ball back to your legs on the next repetition, and keep alternating ball positions for the entire set.

12 repetitions [Advanced]

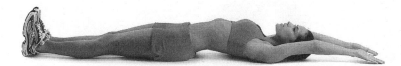

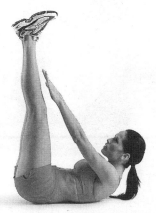

V-UPS
Targets both the upper and lower abs
Lie on your back, with your legs and arms extended. Keeping your knees
and elbows locked, simultaneously raise your upper body while trying to
touch your fingers to your toes.

5–10 repetitions [*Advanced*]

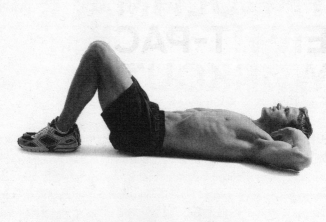

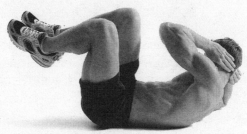

DOUBLE CRUNCH WITH A CROSS

Targets both the upper and lower abs, plus the obliques

Lie on your back with your knees bent, your feet flat on the floor, your head
and neck relaxed, and your hands behind your ears. Use your lower abs to
lift both knees, and cross them towards your left shoulder as you
simultaneously use your upper abs to raise your left shoulder and cross it
towards your right knee. Hold for a second. Lower your legs and torso to the
starting position, and repeat to the other side.

10 repetitions each side [*Advanced*]

BONUS CHAPTER

THE ULTIMATE EIGHT-PACK WORKOUT

New Exercises to Upgrade Your Abs

Why settle for six?

You don't have to be an Olympic gymnast or Bollywood heart-throb to score the ultimate abs trophy – an eight pack. You can sculpt your own in record time if you eat right, add aerobic exercise to your daily regimen, and use the all-new eight-exercise eight-pack programme detailed in this chapter. As you've learned, your abs are actually one long sheet of muscle called the rectus abdominis. Running horizontally across that sheet of muscle are three tendons that hold the muscle in place over the intestines. Another tendon, called the linea alba, divides the rectus abdominis into two parts, creating four pairs of sections. This actually makes the abdomen an eight-pack – not a six-pack, as most people believe. Of course, how easily your eight-pack emerges has to do with genetics, not just diligent effort. Most men have an eight-pack, but weak tendon divisions don't always define the bottom row. If you're one of the lucky ones with taut tendons, you still need discipline to melt the fat that hides the rectus abdominis. And you need to make the abdominal muscles grow by doing advanced exercises that use weights or positions that keep the resistance high and the repetitions low (eight to 15). The pay-off for following this programme is a stronger, more stable core that will help you prevent injury and improve your performance in any sporting activity. This workout has four distinct goals:

Goal 1: A FLAT MID-SECTION!

Most men challenge their midsections with moves that focus primarily on the upper portion of the rectus abdominis, leaving the lower portion overlooked and underdeveloped. That's cheating yourself! Our eight-pack plan gives equal attention to both segments.

Goal 2: MORE SPEED!

The lower abdominals play a crucial role in hip flexion, which moves the knees up and forwards. Training these abs helps you pump your knees higher for longer periods of time, which adds inches to your stride. You'll cover greater distances at faster speeds.

Goal 3: BETTER SKILLS!

When you swing a golfclub or throw a ball, you're channelling power up through your mid-section and into your upper body. Weak abs can cause a break in this transfer of energy. Strong trunk stabilizers transfer the greatest amount of power every time.

Goal 4: STAMINA & BALANCE!

Athletes with weak lower abdominals tend to sway at the waist as they run. This creates additional resistance and forces you to expend extra energy to correct your posture. Strong abs help you maintain the best position for efficiency and extra stamina.

The Workout

Shaping the rare eight-pack requires unique exercises. The smartest way to make your rectus abdominis grow is to perform a mixture of exercises that work your midsection through every possible direction, using as many forms of resistance as possible. These eight exercises incorporate a variety of equipment and partner-assisted moves you may not have tried before.

You'll start your 8-week programme by choosing an exercise from each of the two sections starting on page 280. By the end of the programme, you'll be doing all of them – in the order given – to bring out a level of muscular separation and growth you can't achieve using traditional, high-repetition ab exercises alone. (For the medicine ball and pulley exercises, choose a weight that allows you to do the required number of repetitions with good form. Injuries are common among those who try to speed up results by using more weight than they're ready to handle.)

Time Period

WEEKS 1–2
Create your routine by picking one exercise from each section
Sets of each exercise: 2
Your total workout should be 4 sets
Repetitions per set 8–12
Speed of each repetition: 2 seconds up, 2 seconds down
Rest between sets: 45–60 seconds
Do this workout 3 times a week

WEEKS 3–4
Create your routine by picking one exercise from each section
Sets of each exercise: 3
Your total workout should be 6 sets
Repetitions per set: 8–12
Speed of each repetition: 3 seconds up, 3 seconds down
Rest between sets: 30–45 seconds
Do this workout 3–4 times a week

WEEKS 5–6
Create your routine by picking two exercises from each section
Sets of each exercise: 2
Your total workout should be 8 sets
Repetitions per set: 8–15
Speed of each repetition: 4 seconds up, 4 seconds down
Rest between sets: 15–30 seconds
Do this workout 4 times a week

WEEKS 7–8
Create your routine by doing all the exercises in both sections in the order shown
Sets of each exercise: 1
Your total workout should be 8 sets
Repetitions per set: 8–15
Speed of each repetition: 4 seconds up, 4 seconds down
Rest between sets: None
Do this workout 5 times a week

SECTION 1

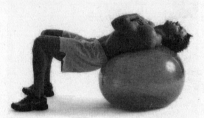

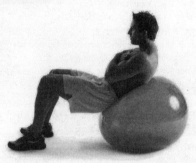

SWISS BALL CURL-UP (UPPER ABS, OBLIQUES)

Recline on a Swiss ball with your head, shoulders, and back in contact with the ball and your feet flat on the floor. Fold your arms across your chest, touching each hand to the opposite shoulder. Pull your belly button in towards your spine to keep your abs tight throughout the move. This helps focus the move more on your abs. Slowly curl your torso up, vertebra by vertebra, stopping just short of an upright-seated position. Then lower yourself to the starting position.

WATCH YOUR FORM: *The ball should not move as you curl.*

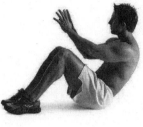

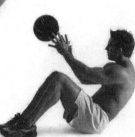

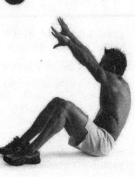

TWISTING MEDICINE BALL TOSS (UPPER ABS, OBLIQUES)

You'll need a partner. Sit on the floor with your hands in front of your chest, knees bent, feet flat on the floor. Your partner should stand a few feet in front of you and to your right. Have your partner toss a medicine ball towards your right side. Catch it and then twist your body to your left, lowering your torso as you go. Touch the ball to the floor, then toss the ball across your body, back to your partner. After a set, reverse the exercise, with your partner throwing the ball from your left.

WATCH YOUR FORM: *As you throw the ball, try to keep your arms straight.*

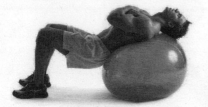

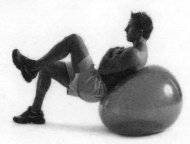

SWISS BALL CURL-UP WITH KNEE TUCK (UPPER AND LOWER ABS, OBLIQUES)

Recline on a Swiss ball, feet flat on the floor, arms crossed on your chest. Your head, shoulders, and back should all be in contact with the ball. Slowly curl your shoulders and upper back up off the ball as you simultaneously draw your left knee towards your chest. Lower your left leg as you lower your torso back down against the ball. Repeat the motion, this time drawing your right knee towards your chest. Continue alternating legs until you've completed all your repetitions.

WATCH YOUR FORM: *Resist the urge to watch your knee move towards your chest.*

V-RAISE (UPPER AND LOWER ABS, OBLIQUES)

Lie on your back with your knees bent at 90 degrees and your feet raised so your thighs are perpendicular to the floor. Slowly extend your legs so they're at a 45-degree angle from the floor as you raise your upper body so your torso is also at 45 degrees. Extend your arms straight out in front of you. Pause, then slowly raise your arms up and back over your head until they're in line with your upper body. Lower your arms so they're parallel to the floor, and return to the starting position.

WATCH YOUR FORM: *If balancing is difficult, raise your arms only as high as you can.*

SECTION 2

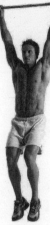

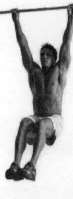

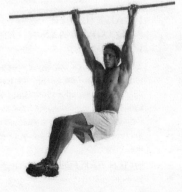

HANGING REVERSE TRUNK TWIST (UPPER AND LOWER ABS, OBLIQUES)

Hang from a pull-up bar with your hands shoulder-width apart and your legs slightly bent. Keeping your legs at this angle, raise them in front of you until your thighs are parallel to the floor. Next, tilt your pelvis and slowly raise your legs until your feet are almost as high as your chest. Lower your legs to the middle position and rotate them to the right (so your feet point to 1 o'clock), then to the left (feet pointing to 11 o'clock). Bring your legs back to the centre, then to the starting position.

WATCH YOUR FORM: *Think about tilting your pelvis up, then lifting your legs.*

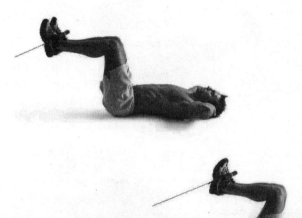

SINGLE-RESISTANCE DOUBLE CRUNCH (UPPER AND LOWER ABS)

Attach a bar to a low-pulley cable. Sit facing the pulley. Place the cable between your feet so that the bar rests across your insteps. Rest your head and back flat on the floor, bend your knees at a 90-degree angle, and position your thighs perpendicular to the floor. Keeping your legs at a 90-degree angle, slowly curl your head and shoulders off the floor as you tilt your pelvis and curl your legs towards your chest. Pause, then return to the starting position.

WATCH YOUR FORM: *Try to curl your lower body forwards to roll your bottom off the floor.*

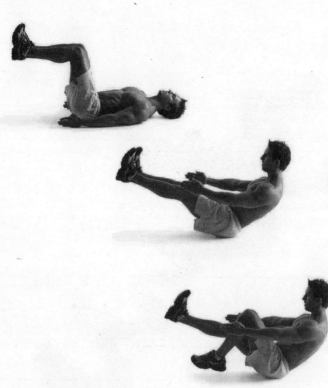

V-RAISE/KNEE TUCK
(UPPER AND LOWER ABS, TRANSVERSE ABDOMINIS)

Lie face-up on the floor with your knees bent at 90 degrees and your feet raised so your thighs are perpendicular to the floor. Slowly extend your legs so they're at a 45-degree angle from the floor and simultaneously raise your upper body so your torso is also at 45 degrees. Extend your arms straight out in front of you. Holding this position, slowly draw your left knee in to your chest, then extend it back out. Repeat the motion with your right leg. Continue to alternate legs.

WATCH YOUR FORM: *Go slowly. Imagine that each foot is resisting something heavy.*

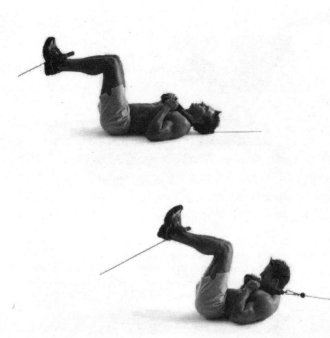

DOUBLE-RESISTANCE DOUBLE CRUNCH (UPPER AND LOWER ABS)

Attach a rope to one of the low-pulley cables and a bar to the other low cable. Lie flat on your back with your head pointing towards the rope and your feet towards the bar. Place the bar on the tops of your shoes so the cable is between your feet. Reach back, grab both ends of the rope, and pull your fists to your chest. Slowly curl your torso up as you simultaneously tilt your pelvis and curl your legs towards your chest. Hold for a second, then slowly lower yourself.

WATCH YOUR FORM: *Try to resist the urge to pull the rope with your arms.*

The Abs Diet Maintenance Plan

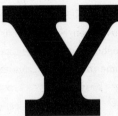**OU'VE REACHED YOUR GOAL, AND** that's reason to celebrate. But it doesn't give you licence to go back to breakfasts of leftover pizza. However, you have earned a reprieve. You've built your body to churn fat and turn it into muscle, and with a muscular base, you're at the point where your body is doing a lot of the work for you. Here's a primer for maintaining the body you've built.

SUBJECT	GUIDELINE
Diet basics	You've adjusted well, and you can continue eating six meals a day by focusing on the Powerfoods – and the super ingredients, like protein, fibre and wholegrain carbohydrates. Keep drinking smoothies regularly and adding a source of protein to every snack.
Cheating	You can up your cheating meal to a cheating day where you treat yourself to anything you want. Just keep it confined to 1 day, rather than spreading it out over several meals on several days. That will increase the chances you'll stay focused and maintain good eating habits.
Exercise programme	You're in maintenance mode now. Keep going with the programme if you like, but you can also scale back to 1 or 2 days a week of strength training and 1 day a week of interval training. Research at the human performance laboratory at Ball State University has shown that weightlifters can maintain their muscle with just one workout a week.
Abdominal workout	Do a circuit of abdominal exercises before your strength training workouts. Move up to advanced exercises. Now that you can see your abs, you will want to increase the intensity. For maximum growth, try the Ultimate Eight-Pack Workout on page 277.

10 Ways to Stick With Your Workout

Funny thing happens when you skip two workouts in a row: You are more likely to skip the next one, and the next after that. We at *Men's Health* magazine have heard all the excuses for skipping exercise. I may have used one or two myself – and didn't feel good about it the next day. But missed workouts do happen. So here's a list of the top reasons that exercise is often pushed to the backburner, whether lame or understandable, and some inspiration from experts who manage to work out no matter how busy their lives become.

First, the legitimate excuses: You're sore, you're sick, you're exhausted, you're hurt. That's it. Soreness means your body needs a break. Overtraining keeps as many men from reaching their goals as under-training does, says Carter Hays, a personal trainer. Take time to allow muscles to recover. An illness means you should knock off and let your body fight the bug. If you're so tired you're drowsy, you could hurt yourself. And if you're injured – especially if you're experiencing joint pain – let your body heal.

As for the rest of the excuses:

I HAVE NO TIME Combine things you do anyway – work, breathe – with athletics. Set up business meetings during which you walk or jog; play tennis with your date; take a spin class to meet people; or take your family hiking, suggests Charles Stuart Platkin, author of *The Automatic Diet*.

LOOKS LIKE RAIN *Men's Health* model Gregg Avedon lives in Florida, home of hurricanes and other tropical storms. So, he spends part of every year lifting storm shutters and storing away patio furniture, then taking cover. He still looks great. Avedon says your home gym – those dumbbells over there, and your chinup bar – makes exercising inside a viable option. You can also spice up your indoor cardio by skipping rope or running up and down stairs.

I DON'T WANT TO SPEND £60 A MONTH ON A GYM MEMBERSHIP Don't. Negotiate fees, trial months, or group discounts. Think you don't have the cash? Save £900 a year by switching from café mocha to metabolism-boosting green tea when you stop at Starbucks every morning.

I'M BORED WITH MY WORKOUT 'Throw it in reverse,' says Gunnar Peterson, author of *G-Force*. If you always do lat pull-downs with an overhand grip, switch to underhand. Do a reverse-grip bench press, reverse-grip curls, reverse-grip triceps pushdowns. Do front squats, rear lunges, and dumbbell lateral raises with your palms up. You can also change to an upper/lower split routine in which you alternate upper-body workouts with lower-body ones. Or try a total-body workout a few times a week.

I HAVE NO ENERGY Eat. You need the fuel. 'An active guy needs up to 1,000 calories more than an inactive guy', says nutritionist Gay Riley.

I CAN'T GET MOTIVATED 'Make an ankle-deep ice-water bath – as cold as you can bear – and stand in it for 20 seconds', says Mark Verstegen, the owner of US studio Athletes' Performance. Then dry off and hit the gym. 'The cold water will shock your nervous system, giving you an immediate rush of energy', he says.

I'M JUST MAKING SURE MY BODY IS GETTING ADEQUATE TIME TO RECOVER After 72 hours of rest, you're just sliding backwards. 'But are you actually giving yourself a chance to recover?' asks Peterson. It's not all about time. Mix L-glutamine into your post-workout shake and eat a diet full of omega-3 fatty acids; they can assist with cellular reconstruction and the removal of metabolic wastes to help you recover faster, Peterson says.

MY MATE CAN'T MAKE IT TONIGHT It's easy to blame others. 'If you're serious about training, think of it like a job', says trainer C. J. Murphy. 'If your training partner was an employee who continually was late and had poor performance, what would you do? You'd sack him!'

EVERYONE'S GOING OUT FOR DRINKS Join them once a week and you won't appear standoffish. But eat first. By having your drinks with a meal, you won't drink, snack and eat dinner later.

I NEED TO WATCH THE KIDS Simplify your workout. Brian Grasso, the CEO of the International Youth Conditioning Association trains all his clients with £25 worth of equipment in his garden. 'We take heavy objects – a wheelbarrow, sandbags or cement bags, for instance – and pick them up, walk with them and lift them overhead. And we use a sturdy tree limb or swing set for pull-ups', he says. Muscle grows best when you train in 'non-linear' patterns, says Grasso. For example, try clockwork push-ups. Keep your feet planted and move around an imaginary clock with your hands, completing 5 push-ups in each position. Another option: Create stations with markers so you can run, jump and skip rope in a variety of patterns. For instance, you might stagger 10 hurdles (boxes, cones, milk cartons) and jump over them 10 times. Then place sticks in an octagonal pattern, stand in the middle of it, and sprint to each corner. You'll slash fat and improve athleticism, all within shouting distance of your family.

In the end, overcoming your excuses just takes a little creativity.

New Abs Diet Recipes: 6-Minute Meals for 6-Pack Abs!

Give Me 6 Minutes for Your Meals, and I'll Give You a 6-Pack for Life

A lot can happen in 6 minutes.

Six minutes is all the time it takes for a Kenyan marathon runner to run more than a mile, and for a rocket headed to Pluto to cover nearly 5,000 miles. Six minutes is the approximate length of some of our careers (think any first-round Apprentice casualty) and some of our marriages ('Welcome back to Las Vegas, Ms Spears!'). Six minutes is enough time to make or break a job interview or have unforgettable sex.

And in 6 minutes, you can find your 6-pack of abs. Let's get it started.

6 Abs Diet Breakfasts

Fire 'em up and start the day strong. What you eat the first hour you're awake will have a huge effect on what you eat for the next 16 or 17. I'm a firm believer that if every day of good eating is a race, then how well you start determines how well you finish.

Quicker Oats

Use plain instant oatmeal for the following recipe. The flavoured instant oatmeal packets contain so much sugar you might as well eat a chocolate bar. Mix all ingredients in a microwave-safe bowl and nuke for 2 minutes, unless otherwise noted. Serves 1.

Honey, I Shrunk My Gut (Powerfoods: 5)

240ml/8 fl oz skimmed milk	1 tsp honey
50g/1¾ oz plain instant oatmeal	1 tsp ground flaxseed (linseed)
100 g/3½ oz blue- or blackberries	Dash of cinnamon
1 tbsp chopped walnuts or pecans	

Per serving: 459 calories; Protein 19 g; Carbs 70 g; Fat 9 g: Saturated fat 2 g; Sodium 132 mg; Fibre 9 g

Flax Machine (Powerfoods: 4)

240ml/8 fl oz skimmed milk

50g/1¾ oz plain instant oatmeal

½ banana, sliced

1 tbsp peanut butter

1 tsp honey

1 tsp ground flaxseed (linseed)

Dash of brown sugar

Per serving: 515 calories; Protein 22 g; Carbs 75 g; Fat 13 g; Saturated fat 3 g; Sodium 172 mg; Fibre 9 g

Instant Omelettes

Omelettes are a quick source of protein – and a chance to boost your Powerfood count with one pan only. For all recipes, stir 2 eggs with a fork until white and yolk are well blended. Add the remaining ingredients. Nuke for 2 minutes and 30 seconds or until the eggs are firmly set. Serves 1.

The Green and White (Powerfoods: 3)

2 eggs

1 tbsp grated low-fat mozzarella cheese

10g/ ½ oz torn baby spinach leaves

Per serving: 221 calories; Protein 15 g; Carbs 3 g; Fat 16 g; Saturated fat 6.5 g; Sodium 256 mg; Fibre 1 g

Bean Counter (Powerfoods: 2)

2 eggs

2 tbsp rinsed black beans

1 tsp coriander

After cooking, top with 1 tbsp salsa.

Per serving: 230 calories; Protein 15 g; Carbs 8 g; Fat 15 g; Saturated fat 6 g; Sodium 361 mg; Fibre 1 g

Breakfast Burritos and Sandwiches

You usually eat burritos for dinner, but a burrito is actually one of the easiest things you can make for breakfast. Just arrange all the ingredients on the tortilla, fold the ends, then neatly roll. For those recipes that call for nuked eggs, you can scramble them in 60 seconds. In a microwave-safe bowl, just stir the eggs with a fork until white and yolk are well blended and microwave for 1 minute per egg.

Huevos Rancheros (Powerfoods: 4)

1 medium whole-wheat tortilla	1 tbsp diced coriander
2 nuked eggs	2 tbsp grated reduced-fat cheese
1 sliced green onion	2 tbsp salsa

Per serving: 326 calories; Protein 20 g; Carbs 25 g; Fat 19 g; Saturated fat 7 g; Sodium 713 mg; Fibre 2 g

The Three-Country Breakfast (Powerfoods: 4)

1 nuked egg	1 toasted whole-wheat English muffin
1 slice lean bacon	1 tbsp shredded reduced-fat cheese
1 slice tomato	

Arrange egg, bacon and tomato on one half of muffin. Top with cheese. Toast in a toaster oven until cheese melts.

Per serving: 326 calories; Protein 24 g; Carbs 30 g; Fat 12 g; Saturated fat 5 g; Sodium 1145 mg; Fibre 5 g

3 Abs Diet Lunches

If there's one meal that you should plan every day, it's lunch. Preparing for it makes you less likely to fall victim to any one of the diet busters waiting to pounce. It doesn't matter whether you make your lunch the night before, in the morning or 3 minutes before you're going to eat it. The point is: Preparation breeds motivation.

Wraps

The trend toward sandwich wraps over the past few years has made eating a healthy lunch easier than ever before. An easy-access tortilla cuts down on empty calories and eliminates the need for utensils. Sticking to your Abs Diet rules, you can create many different healthy wraps for lunches. 1 serving.

The Cow Tipper (Powerfoods: 3)

3 slices roast beef	40g/1¼ oz chopped tomato
1 whole-wheat tortilla	1 tbsp Dijon mustard
50g/1¾ oz mixed greens	1 tbsp blue cheese crumbles

Arrange beef slices down centre of tortilla, then add remaining ingredients. Fold outside edges in, then roll.

Per serving: 208 calories; Protein 22 g; Carbs 26 g; Fat 5 g; Saturated fat 2.5 g; Sodium 1038 mg; Fibre 3 g

Salads

Your standard chain-restaurant salad bar is a nutritional minefield – there are plenty of healthy, safe moves to make and plenty of fat bombs that can blow up your gut: potato salad, macaroni salad, croutons, those bacon bits that look like gravel. If you make your own salad, you can ensure that your salad has taste and power. 1 serving.

Kidney Punch (Powerfoods: 3)

140g/5 oz mixed greens

100g/3½ oz drained tinned kidney beans

1 tbsp chopped onion

Pinch black pepper

1 tbsp red wine

1 tsp olive oil

Per serving: 184 calories; Protein 9 g; Carbs 20 g; Fat 8 g; Saturated fat 2 g; Sodium 154 mg; Fibre 9 g

Pitta Pizzas

Contrary to popular belief, pizza is a health food. The tomato sauce provides vitamin C and the anticancer nutrient lycopene; the cheese gives you a hit of calcium and protein; and any vegetables you toss on top bring extra helpings of vitamins, minerals, and fibre.

Unfortunately, most commercial pizzas are corrupted by excess oil, fatty pepperoni and horrific mutations like 'cheese-filled crust'. Talk about turning a good thing bad!

Try a home version for the taste without suffocating your organs in pepperoni. Spread sauce evenly over pitta, then top with remaining ingredients, you can experiment with different toppings. Bake in an oven preheated to 475°F/245°C/gas 9 for 4 to 6 minutes. Serves 1.

Chicken of the Sea (Powerfoods: 5)

1 small whole-wheat pitta

White sauce (stir together 60 g low fat ricotta cheese, 1 tsp olive oil, ¼ tsp dried basil or oregano)

1 green onion, sliced

1 tbsp low fat mozzarella cheese

45g/1½ oz diced precooked chicken; 1 oz smoked salmon, chopped; or three slices tomato

Chicken: Per serving: 254 calories; Protein 18 g; Carbs 20 g; Fat 12 g; Saturated fat 4.5 g; Sodium 393 mg; Fibre 2 g

Salmon: Per serving: 254 calories; Protein 17 g; Carbs 19 g; Fat 13 g; Saturated fat 5 g; Sodium 827 mg; Fibre 2 g

Tomato: Per serving: 231 calories; Protein 12 g; Carbs 22 g; Fat 11 g; Saturated fat 4.5 g; Sodium 263 mg; Fibre 3 g

6 Abs Diet Dinners

How well you eat at dinner is in great part determined by what you ate earlier in the day. If you fuel your body throughout the day with four smart, sensible meals and snacks, you'll find you aren't ravenously hungry the minute you walk in the door or craving the pulled pork special at O'Bloaty's Tavern. You can, instead, enjoy a hearty – and healthy – meal, either at your favourite restaurant or at home with one of these simple recipes. Instead of using dinner as an opportunity to get drunk on fat and sweets, use it as an opportunity to pack in as many of the POWER 12 as you can.

Burgers

Make yours with lean beef or turkey, grill or broil it just the way you want it, and enjoy a protein blast that will fire up your fat-burners and stimulate muscle growth. Most grocery stores now carry whole-wheat hamburger buns, so your classic 'junk-food' dinner can morph into a perfect diet food – without sacrificing taste.

The Official Abs Diet Burger (Powerfoods: 5)

1 egg	15g/½ oz chopped spinach
1 pound lean ground beef	2 tbsp reduced-fat grated cheese
50g/1¾ oz oats	Salt and pepper
40g/1¼ oz diced onion	

In a large bowl, whisk egg. Add everything else, mixing it – your hands are the best tool – until well blended. Form into four patties. Place burgers in a grill pan or nonstick frying pan that's heated over medium-high. Cook for 6 minutes per side or to desired level of doneness.

Serves 4 (Wrap any extra burgers in plastic and freeze them for later.)

Per serving: 263 calories; Protein 27 g; Carbs 8 g; Fat 13 g; Saturated fat 5 g; Sodium 416 mg; Fibre 1 g

Chicken and Turkey

These two birds are powerful sources of lean protein and great go-to options whenever you're stuck for something to eat. Try these simple concoctions out for size.

The Dijon Lennon (Powerfoods: 3)

2 boneless, skinless turkey cutlets

1 tsp olive oil

80ml/3 fl oz reduced-fat low-sodium chicken broth

1 tbsp Dijon mustard

2 sliced green onions

Salt and pepper to taste

Pound turkey cutlets to an even thickness. Heat oil in nonstick frying pan over medium heat. Brown each side of turkey cutlets, about 3 minutes each. Add broth, mustard, onions, salt and pepper, stirring well. Reduce heat to low. Simmer for 10 to 12 minutes.

Serves 2

Per serving: 140 calories; Protein 27 g; Carbs 2 g; Fat 3 g; Saturated fat 0.4 g; Sodium 364 mg; Fibre 0 g

Gonzo Chicken (Powerfoods: 8)

115g/4 oz bagged mixed-green salad mix

60g/2 oz baby spinach leaves

50g/1¾ oz rinsed chickpeas

90g/3 oz diced precooked chicken

1 tbsp chopped pecans

1 sliced green onion

3 slices avocado

2 tsp olive oil

1½ tbsp balsamic or red wine vinegar

Salt and pepper to taste

Mix greens, chickpeas, chicken, nuts and onion together in a bowl. Top with avocado, oil and vinegar.

Serves 1

Per serving: 420 calories; Protein 30 g; Carbs 27 g; Fat 23 g; Saturated fat 2 g; Sodium 799 mg; Fibre 9 g

Steak

Red meat pulsates with amino acids, the cinder blocks of your body's architecture. In fact, steak is the best natural source of creatine, an enzyme that helps stimulate muscle growth. So unleash your inner carnivore, and you'll unleash your abs as well.

Sergeant Pepper (Powerfoods: 4)

6 ounces flank steak (about half of one)

½ green or red pepper, cut lengthwise into strips

40g/1¼ oz cashew pieces

2 sliced green onions

3 tbsp reduced-sodium soy sauce

Hot sauce, to taste

1tsp sugar

Cut meat diagonally and across the grain into thin strips (freezing it for 20 minutes first helps a lot). Place in large zip-top plastic bag with all other ingredients. Shake well to combine. Place into a pan that's preheated over medium-high heat. Cook for 5 to 6 minutes or until meat reaches desired doneness, turning frequently.

Serves 2

Per serving: 363 calories; 29 g Protein; 14 g Carbs; 22 g Fat; Saturated fat 7 g; Sodium 873 mg; Fibre 1 g

Seafood

Besides delivering plenty of lean protein, most fish are packed with the omega-3 fatty acids that help control cholesterol and your appetite at the same time. To be as sleek and energetic as a dolphin, try this no-hassle recipe.

Hot Pink (Powerfoods: 3)

23-oz cuts of fresh salmon	¼ tsp powdered ginger
1½ tbsp reduced-sodium soy sauce	1 sliced green onion
1 tsp olive oil	1 tsp chopped coriander
Hot sauce to taste	

On a foil-lined pan, place fish on top oven rack under preheated broiler. Broil 4 to 5 minutes or until fish flakes with a fork. Mix soy sauce, olive oil, hot sauce, ginger, onion and coriander in a small microwave-safe bowl. Microwave on high for 5 minutes, stirring once. Remove fish from oven. Transfer to plate, then pour half of the soy sauce mixture over each piece of fish.

Serves 2

Per serving: 203 calories; Protein 20 g; Carbs 1 g; Fat 13 g; Saturated fat 2.5 g; Sodium 460 mg; Fibre 0 g

Pasta

Legend has it that Martin Scorsese took Robert De Niro to Little Italy and directed him to eat pasta in order to balloon up for the second act of Raging Bull. But that doesn't mean you can't eat pasta and still look fighting trim. Whenever possible, opt for the whole-wheat versions; they'll give you gut-filling fibre and help take out a hit on your cholesterol. But with all pasta dishes, the key is to avoid fatty sauces and pile your plate high with Powerfoods.

The Pesto Résistance (Powerfoods: 5)

1 tbsp olive oil	1 tsp dried basil
60g/2 oz walnut pieces	Salt and pepper to taste
1 crushed clove garlic	4 oz whole-wheat spaghetti
60g/2 oz torn baby spinach leaves	2 tbsp grated low fat mozzarella cheese

Heat oil in non-stick pan over medium-low heat. Add nuts and toast 3 to 4 minutes, stirring frequently. Add garlic, spinach, basil, salt and pepper. Cook 3 to 5 minutes more, turning frequently. Toss with cooked pasta and top with cheese.

Serves 2

Per serving: 335 calories; Protein 9 g; Carbs 17 g; Fat 28 g; Saturated fat 4 g; Sodium 160 mg; Fibre 5 g

Index